Economics and Preventing
Healthcare Acquired Infecti

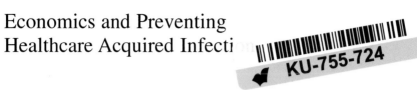

Nicholas Graves • Kate Halton
William Jarvis

Economics and Preventing
Healthcare Acquired Infection

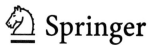 Springer

Nicholas Graves
Queensland University of Technology
Institute of Health & Biomedical Innovation
Musk Avenue & Blamey Street
Kelvin Grove QLD 4059
Australia

Kate Halton
Queensland University of Technology
Institute of Health & Biomedical Innovation
Musk Avenue & Blamey Street
Kelvin Grove QLD 4059
Australia

William Jarvis
135 Dunn Ln
Hilton Head SC 29928-6527
USA

ISBN: 978-0-387-72649-6   e-ISBN: 978-0-387-72651-9
DOI: 10.1007/978-0-387-72651-9

Library of Congress Control Number: 2009926696

Printed on acid-free paper

springer.com

Acknowledgments

We are grateful to the following individuals who gave up their valuable time to read large sections of this book as it was being prepared; they provided excellent comments: Richard Cookson from the University of York; Sonja Firth from Queensland University of Technology; and Jim Zhao from Queensland University of Technology. Linda Robertus worked hard providing supporting material for this project. Our colleagues in Brisbane have supported this project: Michael Whitby and David Cook from the Princess Alexandra Hospital; Dolly Olesen from the Centre for Healthcare Related Infection Surveillance and Prevention; David Paterson from the Royal Brisbane Hospital; Malcolm Faddy, Tony Pettitt, and Adrian Barnett from Queensland University of Technology. We also enjoyed the excellent support of our University managers MaryLou Fleming, Lynne Daniels, and Ross Young.

The preparation of this book was supported by the Queensland Health Quality Improvement and Enhancement Program through the Center for Healthcare Related Infection Surveillance and Prevention.

Contents

List of Figures

List of Tables

List of Panels

Introduction

Reasons for Writing This Book

The published literature on the economic appraisal of healthcare acquired infection (HAI) is described by phrases such as:

> "With so many virtues of the cost-benefit approach identified, it is perhaps puzzling why greater use of economic appraisal has not been made in the area of infection control" [1]

> "Clinicians should partner with economists and policy analysts to expand and improve the economic evidence available" [2]

> "the quality of economic evaluations should be increased to inform decision makers and clinicians" [3]

> "The economics of preventing hospital-acquired infections is most often described in general terms. The underlying concepts and mechanisms are rarely made explicit but should be understood for research and policy-making" [4]

The aim of this book is to describe how economics should be used to inform decision-making about infection control. Our motivation stems from the previous quotes which show economics is being used within the infection control community, but not to its full potential. Our expectation is that you do not have any formal training in economic analyses.

Economic analyses have been used for many decades to argue for increased funding for hospital infection-control. In 1957, Clarke [5] investigated bed wastage in British hospitals due to *Staphylococcus aureus* in patient's wounds. She concluded ....

> "the average length of stay in hospital of patients whose wounds were infected with Staph. aureus was found to be 5 days longer than the average length of stay of patients whose wounds were not so infected"

These are powerful data. The prevention of a case of HAI will free up valuable bed days for alternative uses and so save costs. These savings may compensate the additional expense of an extra infection control program or they may not. There is no doubt, however, that by preventing infection, patients sidestep an event that will affect their quality of life and may even lead to their death. Preventing infections not only changes costs but generates health benefits.

N. Graves et al. *Economics and Preventing Healthcare Acquired Infection.*
DOI: 10.1007/978-0-387-72651-9_1, © Springer Science+Business Media, LLC 2009

There are three mutually exclusive outcomes that follow a decision to implement an infection control program:

Outcome 1. Costly infections are prevented and the cost savings more than offset the costs of achieving them, overall costs decrease. Furthermore, health outcomes improve for patients. This "win win" is rare in today's stressed healthcare environment. Infection control offers the opportunity to save costs while improving health outcomes and no one can argue against that.

Outcome 2. Costly infections are prevented and the savings do not compensate the costs of obtaining them, overall costs increase. Health outcomes improve for patients. Costs are incurred but health benefits are achieved. The value for money of infection control must be compared with other ways of using health care dollars to generate health benefits. Choosing more infection control is better value than some other use of scarce resources, and it should be adopted.

Outcome 3. This is the same as Outcome 2 but infection control is worse value for money than some other alternative, and it might not be adopted. Infection control is not immune from diminishing returns that affect virtually all quality improvement activity. There is almost certainly a point where additional infection control is wasteful and the resources could be used more productively toward some other health goal.

Economics can reveal the best combination of infection control programs while paying attention to alternate ways of spending scarce healthcare dollars. The arguments are relatively simple to make in theory, but implementing economic analyses to change the way a hospital is organized is a challenging task. Demonstrating the economic arguments for good infection control is not trivial and depends on good theory, evidence and supporting data, and some analytic grunt.

The authors of the Study on the Efficacy of Nosocomial Infection Control. (SENIC) project conducted in the 1970s made a positive start. They showed that a good infection control infrastructure that comprised one infection control nurse for every 250 beds, a trained hospital epidemiologist, and feedback of surgical wound infection rates to surgeons had the potential to reduce rates by one third. SENIC also showed that infections imposed economic costs maybe as great as $4.5 billion annually [6] for US hospitals. The economic arguments for good infection control were starting to emerge, but important parts of the jigsaw needed to make compelling arguments were still missing.

Since this time, infection control communities have struggled to develop and communicate the complete economic arguments to policy makers. Reviews of the literature have shown that most studies in the area of economics and HAI describe the costs of HAI only [2, 3]. The infection control community has been served well by these types of studies. Costing studies have placed HAI onto the radarscope of politicians, policy makers, and the press, especially with the rise of MRSA. The range of economic outcomes relevant to infection control is illustrated in Panel 1.

Showing that a disease is costly is not sufficient to complete the economic argument for its prevention [7]. There are four reasons. First, the health benefits that arise from preventing infections are relevant to decision making and must be measured and valued. Costing studies reveal little about the health benefits of prevention programs. Second, preventing cases of HAI is a costly activity itself and these costs are important to decision makers. The adoption of surveillance programs, education programs, and the use of novel devices such as antimicrobial coated central venous catheters are all costly. Studies of the costs of the disease tell us nothing about the costs of preventing the disease. Third, it is unusual to eradicate a disease and this is true of many types of HAI. Costing studies measure the burden arising from the aggregate of all cases of HAI, yet some proportion of these cases can never be avoided. Costing studies tell us nothing about which infections can be prevented and which are inevitable, we therefore do not know exactly which costs will be saved. Fourth, different costs behave in different ways with prevention. Many of the expenditures made for healthcare will not change with lower infection rates in the short term. Costing studies tell us nothing about which costs are fixed and which vary with prevention programs.

Costing studies dominate the infection control literature but are not that useful. A major motivation for writing this book is to describe a framework and method for generating more informative data about the economics of infection control. It is not surprising that good economic analyses have taken a backseat with infection control practitioners and hospital epidemiologists. They are not trained in economic analyses, and the core competencies of a hospital epidemiologist – epidemiology and statistics – are required but not sufficient for the economic analyses. Infection control professionals have faced other challenges including the continued rise of resistant microorganisms, increased levels of morbidity among hospital patients, larger workloads for clinical staff, and constant pressure on hospital productivity. Finding the time to undertake high quality economic analyses of their activities is surely difficult.

Other groups in the healthcare community have, however, used economics to argue for a bigger slice of the pie. For example, population screening for and the treatment of cancer and HIV, and the use of experimental therapies for cardiovascular diseases have all been the subject of high quality cost-benefit and cost-effectiveness studies. These studies have been published in good journals including the New England Journal of Medicine, the Lancet and the Journal of the American Medical Association. Government, regulatory agencies, and others who hold the

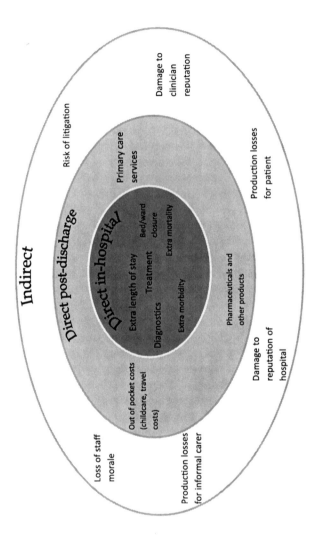

The direct effects of HAI arise during the hospital admission and then after discharge. A patient with an HAI will stay longer in hospital and so use up valuable bed days. They will be diagnosed and treated during the hospital stay which uses up resources. Patients will also feel unwell and some have increased risk of dying from infection, or infection may interact with another symptom to cause premature death. After discharge, patients with infection may use extra health care resources. They may remain on pharmaceutical therapy after discharge and may incur additional out of pocket expenses such as travel costs or child care costs. The indirect effects of HAI include lost production because individuals cannot undertake their normal activities, waged or otherwise, due to the effects of infection. The reputation of the doctors, nurses and hospital may be damaged and the hospital may face litigation.

Panel 1 The range of economic outcomes relevant to infection purse strings for health budgets have been cajoled into funding novel programs based on economic arguments. This is the direction infection control must take. The infection control community must engage with the best research groups, win grants from competitive national funding bodies, publish in good journals and build their research and policy making profile. There is nothing to be gained from circulating the same types of studies, round the same communities, using, by and large, the same research methods, year after year. Infection control must compete with other clinical groups and building strong economic arguments is a good strategy.

The demand for healthcare will continue to rise and spending cannot keep pace. The US economy already devotes one sixth of gross domestic product to health care and many other countries around one tenth. This pressure from cost increases will force the process of choosing the health programs to be funded, and those not to be funded, to become explicit. Professionals working in the area of infection control, which can be relatively cheap and may even save costs, must be ready to justify investment in this area. The methods for making good economic arguments, such as cost-effectiveness analyses, should be part of the infection control professional's toolkit, and this book should be a useful guide.

Audiences for the Book

The audiences for this book are infection control professionals and others interested in adopting infection control programs. The book will serve researchers, practitioners, policymakers, and course tutors. We aim to engage with a clinical audience with little or no training in economics and also hope this book is useful for those who have some experience of health services research, cost-effectiveness, and economic evaluation in health care. We do assume the reader has some knowledge of epidemiology and medical statistics. We propose to take the reader to a basic level of competence in multiple areas but do not claim to be the definitive guide to any single issue. There are specialist research groups with expertise in key areas such as modeling the dynamic nature of disease transmission and the effectiveness of control strategies, predicting the emergence and resource consequences of resistant microorganisms, estimating the complex relationship between HAI and excess length of stay and excess mortality, modeling the effectiveness of infection control programs by synthesizing existing evidence; and modeling risk factors for HAI. Our goal is to stimulate a broad interest in economic analyses, provide a logical framework for thinking about investment decisions and encourage activity among groups who wish to develop research in this area.

The organization of hospital care has many stakeholders with conflicting incentives. The costs and benefits of preventing HAI are voluminous and diffuse. If there were one central cost center that accounted for all the costs and benefits of HAI, then policy making would be easier. Instead, risks are spread across many agents, such as patients, clinicians and the payers of healthcare, and costs range from the minor to the catastrophic. The clever analyst will identify the largest costs and cost savings and health benefits and measure and value them accurately using transparent and rigorous methods. They will then structure the information so the true economic gains from preventing more cases of HAI are unambiguous and the arguments for prevention programs compelling. The natural place for this to happen is in the hospital departments and university research centers inhabited by those who are able to reduce risks of HAI among the hospital population. We hope to lay the foundations for a method for the economic appraisal of HAI. This will reduce the obstacles to high quality research by describing the purpose of economics and health economics and then build knowledge and confidence among readers to develop their own economic analyses.

There are few competitors for this book. Others have published journals articles and book chapters on how to conduct economic analyses for HAI [1, 4, 8–13] but these are constrained to 3,000 words, and this topic is a big one. The authors have to skim across the surface of the topic, or, provide a detailed examination of one part of it. There is duplication among these manuscripts with different definitions and interpretations muddying the waters. We plan to remedy these shortcomings by starting at the beginning, using standard terms and definitions and working through the material in a logical order. Readers will build their knowledge as they progress through the chapters so the material in Chap. 1 will be useful for understanding the ideas presented in Chap. 2 and so on. We use examples and hypothetical data and encourage readers to have a pen, paper, and calculator handy to verify results. This will reinforce understanding.

Organization of the Book

The book is organized into ten chapters. Some readers may be able to dip in and out, using certain chapters to inform certain tasks, but we recommend the reader starts at the beginning and moves forward. The first three chapters can be thought of as a chunk. Together, they set the scene for the rest of the book and lay down some foundations by defining concepts and ways of thinking.

Chapter 1. *Economics:* The discipline is defined and the objectives of economics explained. Six building blocks of economic theory are reviewed and discussed with nontechnical examples. The six building blocks we review are scarcity, opportunity cost, efficiency, competitive markets, market failure and economic appraisal. On first reading, infection control professionals might wonder why they need to learn this material. We believe good economic analyses should rest on strong foundations.

Chapter 2. *Health Economics:* The subdiscipline of health economics is described in this chapter. The work health economists' undertake the parts of health economics likely to be of greatest use for infection control and different approaches to the practice of health economics are described. There are two schools of thought for the part of health economics that will be used extensively in this book, and the differences are fleshed out. We make the decision to jump on board with one school and use this throughout the rest of the book. By the end of the chapter we are ready to start using the techniques of economic appraisal such as cost-effectiveness analysis and cost-utility analysis.

Chapter 3. *Economic Appraisal - A General Description:* We describe in general terms what an economic appraisal looks like and the information required for its successful completion. We consider how the results of an economic appraisal should be used and give examples of correct and incorrect interpretations of the findings.

Chapters 4 and 5 sit together and act as a bridge from the first part of the book which is quite theoretical to the latter chapters which are much more applied.

Chapter 4. *Economic Appraisal - The Nuts and Bolts:* We pick up the pace a little and ask readers to follow the construction of an economic model. We consider how to structure the problem, add data, evaluate the data, and think about uncertainty and its implications for decision making. We finish with a review of the characteristics of a good quality economic appraisal.

Chapter 5. *Changes Arising from the Adoption of Infection Control Programs:* The different types of costs that change with infection control, and how they change are described in this chapter. Costs increase because infection control programs take up resources that need to be funded, but they also save costs because infections, which are themselves costly to deal with, are avoided. Health benefits also increase as infections – that harm patients – are prevented. The methods for measuring the number of infections that might be prevented by some infection control program are also described.

Chapters 6–9 are about how to gather the information required to make the economic arguments for infection control.

Chapter 6. *The costs of Healthcare Acquired Infection:* This chapter is about the best way to measure the costs of HAI. The different way that dollar valuations are attached to resources are described, and this requires some comparison of "cost-accounting" and "economics" methods. The competing epidemiological methods for attributing costs to infection are also reviewed is some detail. We make some recommendations about the best way to estimate the costs of HAI.

Chapter 7. *The Costs of Infection Control Programs:* The measurement and interpretation of the costs of implementing infection control programs are considered in this chapter. Two case studies are presented. We use data in both tabular and graphical form to show how costs might be estimated and then interpreted.

Chapter 8. *Preventing HAI and the Health Benefits that Result:* This chapter is about the health benefits that arise from preventing cases of infection. Both the quality of life gains (avoided ill health) and the quantity of life gains (avoided death) are covered. The methods for describing and then valuing the health benefits from preventing infections are described. To make the complete economic argument, the health benefits that arise from preventing HAI are just as important as any change to cost outcomes from prevention.

Chapter 9. *Dissecting a Published Economic Appraisal:* In this chapter, a published economic evaluation of using antimicrobial catheters to reduce the risks of catheter-related bloodstream infection is dissected. So far we have used lots of hypothetical examples and convenient case studies to make our points. In this chapter, the gloves come off, and we talk you though a real economic appraisal – warts and all – to illustrate that conducting this type of research is possible but at times complex and involved. Chapter 9 is a biggie and we recommend two sittings, with a walk round the block in between, to reduce the chance of indigestion.

Chapter 10. *Role of Economics in the Infection Control Environment:* The final chapter is an exposition of how economics can be used at the coal face of infection control. Some important challenges faced by infection control professionals are analyzed using the material that has been developed in the previous chapters. We draw our conclusions, tie the ideas together, and provide a summary of the whole book.

We hope you enjoy reading this book and that it allows you to look at infection control from a different perspective. We cannot hope to turn you into health economist. If that is your goal you should enroll in a masters or PhD health economics program. That would be a wonderful contribution as there are few people with health economics working in this field. If we can stimulate your thinking and spark an interest in the use of economic analyses to improve infection control arrangements then we have done our job.

Chapter 1
Economics

Preview

- The aim of this chapter is to introduce the reader to economics.
- The discipline of economics is defined and the objectives explained.
- Six building blocks of economic theory are reviewed.
- We believe that a good economic analysis of infection control should rest on strong foundations.

1.1 A Broad View of Economics

An economic system – big or small – must select and then structure its activities. It might be a national economy or a medium size hospital, but three key questions are the same:

  (i) *What* should be done?
 (ii) *How* should it be done?
(iii) *Who* will enjoy the benefits of the chosen activities?

Economics is concerned with answering these questions.

A national economy such as the United States or the United Kingdom is the sum of its resources, which fall in two groups, capital and labor. Capital resources include land, fossil fuels, buildings, computers, heavy machinery, brand names and reputation. Labor is the time individuals spend working, whether waiting on tables, cleaning or clerical work, or in more structured professions such as accountancy, architecture, or medicine. How capital and labor resources are used define an economy. This is important because resources are finite, yet there are many different ways to use them. Getting it wrong and making bad choices about how to use scarce resources can lead to great hardship and poverty. Successful economies, where resources have been allocated with some efficiency, deliver a good standard of living for the majority of the population.

A medium size hospital is also the sum of its resources. It comprises capital resources, from diesel generators to surgical robots, and many different types of labor, from cooks to cardiologists. Those who manage hospitals have to think long

N. Graves et al., *Economics and Preventing Healthcare Acquired Infection*,
DOI: 10.1007/978-0-387-72651-9_2, © Springer Science + Business Media, LLC 2009

and hard about how they use resources because like those of national economies, resources are finite and can be used in many different ways. Making bad choices about how to allocate a hospital's resources between competing activities can cause worse health outcomes for patients.

We have decided that cracking nuts is a useful activity that we wish to devote scarce resources to. We have a budget of $20 (our scarce resources) that can be used to acquire a hammer or a nut cracker in order to complete the task. Using our scarce resources to buy the nut cracker provides more benefits than if we had chosen the hammer.

Making good choices about how to allocate scarce resources is central to economics. We have decided that cracking nuts is a useful activity that we wish to devote some scarce resources to. We have a budget of $20 (our scarce resources) that can be used to acquire a hammer or a nut cracker in order to complete the task. Using our scarce resources to buy the nut cracker provides more benefit than if we had chosen the hammer. It is faster and achieves a better outcome. The best decision is one that maximizes benefit from the resources available. As long as you understand this, you are starting to think like an economist.

Economists work with politicians, business people, lawyers, and academics to allocate resources that make-up an economic system, to obtain the best value or benefits for society. The aim of economics is to make the maximum number of people as happy as possible, given finite resources. To achieve this requires careful consideration of those three key questions:

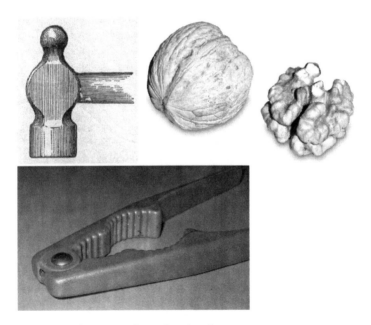

Fig. 1 Two ways to crack a nut, one better than the other

 (i) *What* should be done?
 (ii) *How* should it be done?
 (iii) *Who* will enjoy the benefits of the chosen activities?

Economics is used in two ways. *"Positive Economics"* explains *what actually happens* in society. It answers "what is" type questions, such as, "What is the effect of allocating scarce resources in order to host the Olympic Games?," *"Normative Economics,"* on the other hand, is used to identify *what should happen.* It answers questions about "what ought to be," such as whether the Olympic Games should be hosted. Is it more valuable to society than some other use of scarce resources, such as poverty relief or improved access to healthcare? Normative questions stimulate debate because they require value judgments to be made. Positive decisions are less contentious because they are based on facts. Both forms of economics are concerned with the study of how resources are allocated within an economic system. This book is concerned with how resources are used for the purpose of infection control. This implies that both positive and normative questions will be addressed. We need to gather facts about what infection-control might cost and what benefits it may provide, yet we also need to make judgments on how valuable those outcomes are compared with other ways of using scarce healthcare resources. This book is a mixture of positive and normative economics.

   Some economic concepts that will be useful throughout this book are described in the next section. These are Scarcity, Opportunity Cost, Efficiency, Competitive Markets, Market Failure, and Economic Appraisal. Our objectives are to define these terms using nontechnical language, bring them together like building blocks and encourage you to think like an economist. Economics is useful if you want to show why something should change. This book is about preventing healthcare-acquired-infections and we aim to provide readers with enough economics to make rational and well constructed arguments about why something should change with the current allocation of infection-control resources. You can make your economic arguments to a middle manager in your hospital or the chief executive, local or regional health planners, or state or national politicians. The principles and arguments remain the same and are quite simple. You may wish to argue for more resources to be devoted to infection-control and away from some other activity, or for existing infection-control resources to be used in another way. We offer you a set of tools and a way of thinking that can improve how decisions are made and, ultimately, how scarce resources are used for infection control.

1.2 The Building Blocks of Economics

1.2.1 The Concept of Scarcity

Scarcity is at the core of economics. Not all of societies' objectives can be achieved with the available resources. Although it might be desirable to improve education and healthcare services, this would require cuts to some other part of the economy, such as law enforcement or road maintenance. Every household might like to have a new car and three foreign holidays a year, but this might require cuts to mortgage payments or retirement savings. Scarcity arises because humans have a voracious desire to be successful. Some want material goods, big houses, and sports cars; others desire recognition in the community and want to help others; while some may just desire a simple but comfortable life in the countryside. However, the capital and labor resources required to make all these things happen are finite.

Hadley Cantril [14] collected some data that illustrate the range of human wants. The people interviewed lived in India or the United States, and here are some extracts:

India – 35-year-old man, illiterate, agricultural laborer.

I want a son and a piece of land... I would like to construct a house of my own and have a cow for milk and ghee. I would also like to buy some better clothing for my wife. If I could do this then I would be happy.

India – 45-year-old housewife.

I should like to have a water tap and a water supply in my house. It would also be nice to have electricity. My husband's wages must be increased if our children are to get an education and our daughter is to be married.

United States – 34-year-old laboratory technician.

I would like a reasonable enough income to maintain a house, have a new car, have a boat, and send my four children to private schools.

United States – 28-year-old Lawyer.

Materially speaking, I would like to provide my family with an income to allow them to live well - to have the proper recreation, to go camping, to have music and dancing lessons for the children, and to have family trips. I wish we could belong to a country club and do more entertaining.

These individuals all strive for more. They reveal material and social aspirations for themselves and their families (i.e., a cow, tap water, a boat, or dancing lessons); the difference is that some have more resources than others and so prefer different things. Most Americans take running water, electricity, and a house for granted, yet these extracts reveal that this is not the case in India. The argument we make is that humans always want more of something, regardless of the circumstances.

John Maynard Keynes is the father of macroeconomics and made a prediction in the 1930s. He suggested increases in wealth would lead to a situation where individuals would have all their needs (demands) met and so would cease to strive for more of anything, instead devoting further energies to "noneconomic purposes" [15]. The examples of Imelda Marcos and her enthusiasm for shoes and Jay Leno and his passion for motoring, suggest otherwise. Human wants will never be fully satisfied, and because resources are finite, choices will always have to be made about how they are used.

The more productively resources are used the more goods and services are available. The result is that citizens of some countries have more material possessions than others. The American and Indian economies are both rich in resources, yet the American economy extracts more value from available resources when compared

| Jay Leno is a car enthusiast with an impressive collection of modern and vintage vehicles. The collection is always growing, even though he can only drive one at a time. | In 1986 Imelda Marcos and her husband fled the Philippines after a revolution against a corrupt regime. She left behind mink coats, 508 gowns, 888 handbags and 1060 pairs of shoes. |

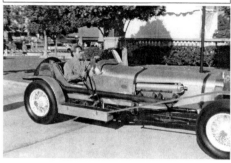
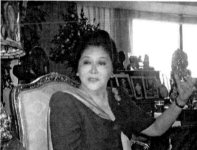

with the Indian economy. This difference will diminish if the Indian economy continues to grow rapidly. Decisions are made everyday in both countries about what can and what cannot be done with scarce resources, and this is because of scarcity. Scarcity is the core of economics.

Paul Samuelson wrote this definition of economics [16],

> *"economics is the study of how men and society end up choosing, with or without the use of money, to employ scarce productive resources that could have alternative uses, to produce various commodities and distribute them for consumption, now and in the future, among various groups in society"*

He goes on to describe the three challenges for any economy.

Challenge One: *What* commodities shall be produced and in what quantities?

Challenge Two: *How* should they be produced?

Challenge Three: *Who* will enjoy the benefits of the commodities?

The process of answering these questions will give rise to an allocation of resources. It is important to answer these questions as appropriately as possible. Because of scarcity, when a choice is made, an opportunity to do something else is lost and this is called an opportunity cost.

1.2.2   The Concept of Opportunity Cost

We cannot do everything we want (think about scarcity), and a decision to use resources in one way causes a loss elsewhere in the economy. The loss arises because resources are no longer available for an alternative use. If a hospital manager decides to screen every new admission for methicillin-resistant *Staphylococcus aureus* (MRSA), then some resources would be used up. These include *labor resources*, such as the time of doctors, nurses, microbiologists, and infection-control professionals, and *capital resources*, such as isolation beds, gowns, gloves, microbiology equipment, and other consumables. Without the screening program, these resources could have been used to treat 500 new patients. The benefits from treating these extra patients represent the opportunity costs of the MRSA screening program. How these opportunity costs are valued depend on the perspective of the analyst. The hospital manager would look at the financial revenues foregone from not admitting the 500 new patients. A public health professional might estimate the years of life saved from diagnosing and treating the symptoms of the 500 patients. These two estimates are mutually exclusive. We cannot count the lost financial revenues to the hospital and the years of life lost, which would be double-counting. However, we could attempt to attach a dollar figure to the years of life lost and represent dollar estimates of opportunity costs this way. Economists tend to think about broader social objectives when making suggestions about how resources should be used and would therefore prefer the second approach to estimating opportunity costs.

There are situations where the opportunity cost of a decision is zero, or close to it. If there were no new patients waiting to be admitted to the hospital, staff were protected by long-term employment contracts and so could not be released, and if there was a stock of consumables that had to be used before an imminent expiry date, then the opportunity costs of the MRSA screening program would be zero. The reason is that the resources could not be used in another way and so no benefits have been foregone by deciding to screen for MRSA. If there were no patients waiting to be admitted but the resources could be turned into cash by firing staff and selling the consumables to another hospital, then the cash generated would represent the opportunity cost of the MRSA screening program.

The United States administration of the early 1960s made a decision to send man to the moon and return him safely to the earth. This project used billions of dollars worth of scarce resources and was built on the vision of Werner Von Braun, an active member of the "Society for Spaceship travel" in 1930s Germany. An economist would ask what else could have been done with the resources. On the brink of the launch of Apollo 11, powered by the Saturn rocket illustrated in Fig. 2, Reverend Ralph Abernathy led a march of the Poor People's Campaign to Cape Canaveral to make exactly this point. He spoke with Thomas Paine, the NASA administrator at the time, and suggested the opportunity costs of the Apollo program were great, highlighting the poverty and suffering in American society. He argued poverty and suffering could be reduced with a reallocation of resources away from space exploration and toward interventions that reduce the causes and consequences of poverty. Whether Reverend Abernathy had a good economic argument depends on the value of the Apollo program relative to a poverty alleviation program or any other competing uses of scarce resources.

Some made-up data that describe the benefits of the Space program and the competing alternative ways of using scarce resources are included in Table 1.

Interpreting these data is quite simple. We choose the alternative that provides the greatest net benefit. Because we are constrained by scarcity, we only have enough resources to implement one program, and all programs use the same amount of resources. The decision to choose one program implies a loss, as we have rejected the others. The value of this loss is the opportunity cost. The decision to choose the space program implies a loss of benefits from poverty alleviation and these are valued

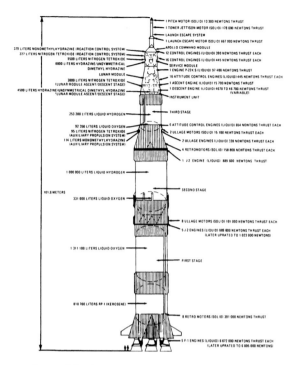

Fig. 2 The Saturn rocket used for the space program that put man on the moon

Table 1 An example of opportunity cost

Options	Description of the economic benefits	Dollar valuation of economic benefits[a]
Space Program	Scientific advances Commercial spin offs Cold war supremacy Extending frontiers	$150 billion
Poverty Alleviation	Improved health Reduced crime Better workers Increased tax revenue	$120 billion
Tax cuts for the wealthy	Increased savings Increased spending Increased luxury car sales Increased overseas travel	$60 billion

[a] We assume that estimating the dollar values for economic benefits is easy. In reality, it is difficult and requires normative judgments to be made. Economists and policy makers argue long and hard about how to value things that are not traded in competitive markets (i.e., easy to acquire from shops or other suppliers), and these debates have shaped how economic analyses are structured and undertaken

at $120 billion. This is the opportunity cost of the space program. As the decision to pursue the Space program provides benefits worth $150 billion then we are better off by $30 billion.

The complete decision is summarized like this:

> Space program: Benefits of $150 bn less opportunity costs of $120 bn = positive $30bn

> Poverty Alleviation: Benefits of $120 bn less opportunity costs of $150 bn = negative $30bn

> Tax cuts for the wealthy: Benefits of $60 bn less opportunity costs of $150 bn = negative $90bn

The space program delivers positive net benefits of $30 billion and the other two options necessarily incur net losses. Take a little time to make sure you understand this. This conclusion leads to a simple decision-rule that requires only those activities that provide the maximum difference between benefit and cost to be chosen, given scarce resources. This is equivalent to making decisions that maximize net benefit. We prefer to allocate scarce resources to programs that maximize net benefit because all members of society can be made better off. Those who enjoy the economic benefits can cover all the costs, and there is enough left over to compensate everyone else. If we choose a program that leads to losses, then there is no way to finance the program without leaving some people worse off. If this rule is applied to all possible decisions in society, then the maximum amount of benefit will be generated.

We now consider an example from the hospital setting. The management board has resources available to implement one of three programs: MRSA screening, the purchase of a surgical robot, or an upgrade to the hospital information technology (IT) system. Data on the benefits of these programs are summarized in Table 2.

Table 2 An example of opportunity cost relevant to infection control

Competing decisions	Description of the economic benefits	Dollar valuation of economic benefits[a]
MRSA screening	Reduced rate of infection Shorter length of stay Reduced mortality	$100,000
Surgical robot	Better surgical outcomes Shorter procedure duration Reduced mortality	$60,000
Upgrade to the hospital IT system	Improved user interface More accurate billing Link to primary care records	$48,000

[a]Valuing the economic benefits from healthcare is also difficult. Lives may be at risk and so the consequences of decisions are potentially devastating to those involved. The methods for valuing a human life are important for health economics and these are described at the end of this chapter

The application of the decision rule suggests net benefits of the "MRSA screening" program are $100,000 less $60,000 opportunity costs = positive $40,000 and so choosing one of the other alternatives will lead to net losses (i.e., the robot has $60,000 benefit less $100,000 opportunity costs which equals losses of $40,000, and the IT system has $48,000 benefit less $100,000 opportunity costs which equals losses of $52,000). Opportunity costs have been calculated by identifying the value of the benefits foregone with each decision. With this information we would always choose MRSA screening. The surgeon and users of the IT system who have incurred a loss will have to be placated, but decisions are made on behalf of the whole community. The adoption of the space program and the MRSA screening program enhance efficiency by the allocation of scarce resources.

1.2.3   The Concept of Efficiency

Economics is about scarcity, opportunity cost, and using resources such that benefits to society are maximized. Improvements in an economic system need to be measured, be it a whole country or a single hospital, and for this we use a yardstick called economic efficiency. Economists are nearly always interested in improving economic efficiency. Economic efficiency is about choosing the optimal use (i.e., allocation) of scarce resources. An economic system is said to be economically efficient when scarce resources are used to produce the maximum amount of goods and services that individuals want. Two conditions must be met before economic efficiency can be achieved. These are "allocative" and "productive" efficiency. The concepts are illustrated by Fig. 3.

Allocative efficiency is when producers choose to produce the right goods and services, they are *"doing the right things."* We used hypothetical data to show that the Space Program and MRSA screening were the right things to do. Productive efficiency is when producers make these goods at minimum cost; they are *"doing things right."* Those who organized the Space program and the MRSA screening must pursue these activities at minimum costs and waste nothing. For example, MRSA screening could be done at a routine preadmission clinic, or a separate consultation could be organized and a dedicated MRSA nurse employed to perform the swabs. The former is likely to be more productively efficient (cheaper) than the latter.

Vilfredo Pareto was a well known philosopher and economist who died in 1923. His interpretation of economic efficiency was an allocation of resources where no individual can be made better off without another being made worse off, from any further reallocation. A balance has been reached where scarce resources are being used to produce the maximum amount of goods and services that people want. To achieve this outcome, decisions like those to adopt the space or MRSA screening programs would have to be made until no further gains were possible from scarce resources. The winners from the space program would have received net benefits worth $30 billion and according to Vilfredo Pareto, they must compensate every-

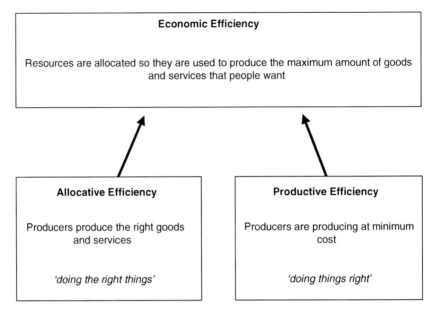

Fig. 3 Three types of efficiency

body else. The $30 billion profit is the reason we chose the "Space program" in the first place. The other programs would have left us worse off. The winners from the MRSA screening program enjoyed benefits worth $40,000, and they would have to compensate everyone else who missed out. Again, the $40,000 profit is why we chose MRSA screening.

Making these compensations in reality is difficult and so economists suggest the compensations do not actually have to happen, but instead only the possibility for compensation has to exist. This rule, known as the Kaldor-Hicks criterion, is not perfect, but it does add flexibility to decision making and oils the cogs of economic efficiency. The rule allows decisions to be made where some individuals are winners and others are losers; furthermore, the winners do not actually have to compensate the losers, they just have to be able to make the compensations.

There are two mechanisms in an economy that influence resource allocation under scarcity. The first is the use of "Competitive Markets" and the second is the use of "Economic Appraisal." Because these two mechanisms inform resource allocation, they impact on efficiency. The workings of the market and the process of economic appraisal are the subjects for the remaining sections of this chapter.

1.2.4   The Concept of Competitive Markets

A market can be used to allocate scarce resources and so address the three key questions for an economic system. Markets encourage infinite cost-benefit calculations amongst all those who participate, just the same as were done to choose the space program and the MRSA screening programs. A market is a physical or virtual environment where producers and consumers interact. A fruit and vegetable market held in the local park every Saturday morning is an example of a physical market, and the global market for iron ore is a virtual market as you do not have to be physically present to participate. The role of a market is to allow producers and consumers to exchange goods and services. It is driven by the rule of maximizing net benefits and has the desirable outcome of allocating scarce resources efficiently. Consumers demand goods and services in a market, and every consumer knows exactly how valuable the items are. Producers learn about what consumers want (i.e., demand), and then meet those demands by allocating scarce resources to productive processes. Consumers are "sovereigns" as they ultimately decide how producers use scarce resources. The market is an environment that disciplines producers into making things that enhance economic efficiency. A producer who allocates scarce resources to manufacturing goods and services that consumers do not value the most will be fail in the market.

The Sinclair C5 illustrated here suffered the wrath of the market. Although some might say this product was ahead of its time, the consumers of 1985 were not impressed with this plastic, battery-powered single-seater. A journalist who tested this vehicle concluded:

> *"I would not want to drive a C5 in any traffic at all. My head was on a level with the top of a juggernaut's tyres, the exhaust fumes blasted into my face. Even with the minuscule front and rear lights on, I could not feel confident that a lorry driver so high above the ground would see me. Small wonder that one of the accessories listed in the C5 brochure is a high and bright-red reflecting mast."*

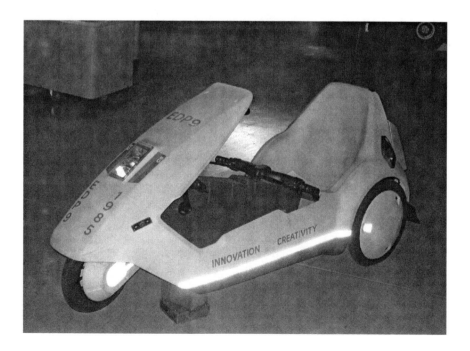

Only 12,000 were produced and very few were demanded by consumers. The C5 was a commercial disaster. Consumers exerted their sovereignty, signaled that the C5 was not going to increase economic efficiency and ensured no more resources were allocated to its production.

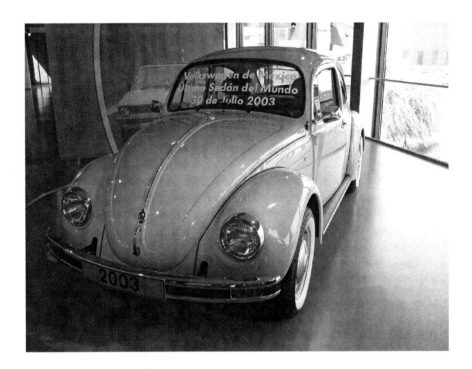

In contrast, consumers loved the Volkswagen Beetle. Demand was strong for this cheap, reliable, and quirky car from 1938 to 2003, when production in Mexico finally ended. The less popular but more beautiful VW Karmann Ghia was a success too. Consumers sent signals to producers about what to make and how to make it. This allocation of resources (away from C5s and toward Volkswagens) was made by the *"invisible hand"* of the market [17].

Adam Smith first used this phrase – the invisible hand – in 1776 to argue that the goods and services of most benefit to society will, naturally, also be those that are most attractive for producers. The force behind the invisible hand is the price system, which is at the heart of a competitive market. The data included in Fig. 4 demonstrate how the price system works. If the price of a physical item or service is $5, then consumers in the market only demand one item. They seek alternate ways of obtaining benefits from their scarce resources in other markets. Yet, at $5, producers want to make five units because the price is high and they can make good money. This market is out of balance as there is a surplus of four unsold items. Consumers are busy spending their money in other markets where they get better value for money.

WHEN THE PRICE IS:	THIS QUANTITY IS:			THERE IS A MISMATCH OF:
	wanted	*offered*	*traded*	
$5	I	IIIII	I	surplus of IIII
$4	II	IIII	II	surplus of II
$3	III	III	III	zero: market in balance
$2	IIII	II	II	shortage of II
$1	IIIII	I	I	shortage of IIII

Fig. 4 How the price system works

When the price is only $1, consumers want five items because they are now represent good value for money, yet producers only want to produce one item because of the small profit at the low price. The market is again out of balance, and there is a shortage of four items. Producers are busy using their resources to produce goods and services that can be sold in more profitable markets. Because of this shortage, consumers now bid against each other for the item and the price rises. This will stimulate producers to allocate resources toward production, as they see profits at higher prices. When the price reaches $3, both parties are satisfied and the market has reached a balance. The price tells consumers how to spend their money, and the producers follow this lead by making what the consumers want in exactly the way they want it. If every consumer is allowed to choose what they buy and producers are allowed to choose what to produce, then the market will find the balance. This is an allocation of resources that produces the maximum amount of goods and services that individuals want and represents a state of economic efficiency.

Joseph E. Stiglitz [18] summarizes these ideas:

> If there is some commodity or service that individuals value but that is not currently being produced, then they will be willing to pay something for it. Entrepreneurs, in their search for profits, are always looking for such opportunities. If the value of a certain commodity to a consumer exceeds the cost of production, there is a potential for profit, and an entrepreneur will produce that commodity. Similarly, if there is a cheaper way of producing a commodity than that which is presently employed, an entrepreneur who discovers this cheaper method will be able to undercut competing firms and make a profit. The search for profits on the part of entrepreneurs is thus a search for more efficient ways of production and for new commodities that better serve the needs of consumers.(pp. 56–57)

Perfectly competitive markets seem a very smart way to allocate scarce resources. Economic efficiency is achieved, net benefits maximized in society and scarce resources are used efficiently. The first two questions of economics, (i) *what* should be done and (ii) *how* should it be done, have been addressed. The third question, (iii) *who* will enjoy the benefits of the activities, is also addressed because consumers express their preferences for certain goods and services in markets.

In a perfect world, the initial distribution of wealth is fair with an extra dollar of benefit valued equally by any member of society, for example, a poor American living in rural Kansas would value another dollar exactly the same as would the chief executive of a large company building fuel tanks for the Saturn rocket. In the real world (the not-perfect world), the wealthy place a lower value on an extra dollar than the poor, and this poses problems when we use efficiency as a criterion for making decisions and deciding how resources are allocated. Some economists believe that economic efficiency and questions of how wealth is distributed should be dealt with separately, the former by economists and the latter by politicians. Politicians control the mechanisms for redistributing income, which are taxes, subsidies, and government ownership of certain industries. For our purposes, we make the simplistic assumption that government policy will lead to a fair distribution of wealth and so focus on economic efficiency.

If resource allocation is so easy using competitive markets, why is economics still practiced so widely? The answer is that markets do not always work and often fail to find an efficient allocation of resources. The causes of market failure are the next topic.

1.2.5 The Concept of Market Failure

A market will fail to find an efficient allocation of scarce resources for a number of reasons: market power, external costs and benefits, and the nature of certain goods and services.

Market Power: It is very important that no-one gains control of the market. Perfect competition relies on having many consumers and producers in the market. This ensures that every individual consumer and producer is a negligible part of the market and so has no power over how the market functions. If there are many small producers, it is hard for them to collude and increase the price above the natural market price. Producers must accept the market price. If there are many consumers then it is difficult for them to organize themselves to manipulate the price downwards. Also, every product traded must be identical in every way (i.e., homogenous). The rule of perfect competition encourages producers to compete on price alone and so minimize costs. Any deviation from perfect competition is likely to lead to an inefficient allocation of resources.

External costs and benefits: The supply of some goods and services in a market cause costs or benefits that impact on others and these are called externalities. The owners of a chemical plant who pollute the local water supply impose costs on others and the use of antibiotics may impose costs on others by causing resistant organisms to develop. These are both negative externalities. The converse are positive external benefits such as the occurrence of herd immunity arising from a vaccination program or the provision of a work-based keep fit program that encourages individuals to ride or walk to work and so parking becomes easier for those who have to drive. The presence of good and bad externalities will fool the market into an inefficient allocation of scarce resources.

*The nature of some goods and services:*Some goods and services are "public goods," which cannot be traded in perfectly competitive markets. Public goods are those that jointly benefit many people, yet it is difficult to exclude individuals from. An example is national defense. If scarce resources are allocated to defending a country, then the entire population is protected. It is impossible to select protection for some individuals and exclude others. For this reason, it is difficult to find out how individuals value the benefits of defense and without this information perfectly competitive markets cannot function. There are also goods and services that are not public goods that consumers still find difficult to value. For markets to work properly, consumers and producers must understand the quality, attributes, and prices in the market, so they know what they should buy to make themselves happy. Poor information may lead to mistakes and a failure to choose an efficient mix of goods and services. Information deficits can be remedied using an expert agent who has good knowledge of the product. An honest and hard working car mechanic will fulfill this role. This agency relationship can be problematic as the agent can induce the consumer to demand more of a good than they might have wanted if they had had perfect information. A dishonest car mechanic might convince you to refit a brake system that in reality will be perfectly safe for another 5,000 miles. This would not be an efficient outcome as you will have incurred positive cost and zero benefit.

Healthcare, including infection control, falls foul of most of these requirements [13]. It is very unlikely that we can use markets to allocate scarce resources efficiently. Healthcare is an unusual good. For a start, no consumer actually wants healthcare, few people enjoy visiting hospital and being jabbed, poked, or chopped up. Lance Armstrong is a cancer survivor who has won the Tour de France many times. He made the following description of what it is like to demand healthcare:

> "One thing they don't tell you about hospitals is how they violate you. It is like your body is no longer your own, it belongs to the nurses and doctors, and they are free to prod you and force things into your veins and various openings. The catheter was the worst; it ran up my leg into my groin, and having it put in and taken out again was agonizing. In a way, the small, normal procedures, were the most awful part of illness. At least for the brain surgery I'd been knocked out, but for everything else, I was fully awake, and there were bruises and scabs and needle marks all over me, in the backs of my hands, my arms, my groin. When I was awake the nurses ate me alive."(REF)

Consumers are unlikely to value the process of healthcare, but they do value the end product, improved health, and what that allows them to achieve in life, yet scarce resources are used to produce healthcare. There is a difference between health and healthcare, and the demand for healthcare services is derived from a demand for health. This is not a good start if we want to use perfectly competitive markets to decide how scarce resources are used in healthcare.

There are further problems. Producers often have market power in healthcare. Doctors tend to restrict entry to the medical profession by limiting the places available in medical schools and any healthcare professional must obtain the appropriate experience, qualifications, certifications, and licenses – for good reasons – before they enter the market. This means that consumers cannot always pick and choose who they purchase their goods and services from and healthcare producers often enjoy a monopoly; this is the opposite of perfect competition. Healthcare is not homogenous, everyone is slightly different and so producers can discriminate between consumers, robbing them of their collective bargaining power. With monopoly producers and many different products in the market, prices will tend to be higher than a competitive market would allow and this is not efficient. Healthcare markets are characterized by positive and negative externalities leading to further inefficiency in resource allocation and parts of health care are public goods, such as effective antibiotics. If we left the supply of antibiotics to the competitive market (as has happened in parts of south-east Asia), then the negative externality of antibiotic resistance would be ignored by the market, and this results is a poor allocation of resources. Consumers also lack information in health care markets. They will not know when they need healthcare, and after they get sick they will not know what's wrong with them, how to treat it, or whether they will prefer an aggressive treatment or some other approach. Instead, they rely on doctors and other healthcare professionals to express their demand for healthcare via an agency relationship. The advent of Health Maintenance Organizations (HMOs) in the United States offers more bargaining power over doctors on behalf of consumers, but the situation is still a long way from the perfect market.

It is unlikely that economic efficiency will be achieved via perfectly competitive markets in healthcare. Without the invisible hand to guide resource allocation, the costs and benefits of different decisions, and so the opportunity costs, must be measured manually. The process by which the costs and benefits of different uses of scarce healthcare resources is measured is called economic appraisal.

1.2.6   The Concept of Economic Appraisal

Economic appraisal is the manual collection of the information that competitive markets provide so effortlessly. We have seen that perfectly competitive markets gather all this information with apparent ease. Tim Harford, author of the Undercover Economist [19], describes the perfect market as:

> "a giant supercomputer network. With amazing processing power and sensors in every part of the economy – reaching even inside our brains to read our desires – the market is constantly reoptimising production and allocating the results perfectly"

Economic appraisal is what must happen when the supercomputer keeps crashing because of market failure. In the case of healthcare, the market will not work, and so the hard calculations about costs, benefits, and what is efficient to produce have to be made manually with a slide-rule and abacus. Economic appraisal is, therefore, used to help decision makers allocate scarce resources between competing alternatives when market mechanisms fail. This chapter began with two examples of economic appraisal. The evaluation of the costs and benefits of the "space program" vs. two other alternatives, and the evaluation of the costs and benefits of an "MRSA screening program" vs. two alternatives provided information about how resources might be allocated to improve efficiency.

One of the hardest parts of economic appraisal is to value the economic benefits of one activity over another. The competitive market requires consumers to reveal their valuations of the benefits of various goods and services relative to all other choices. When markets do not work, benefits have to be valued manually, and this is difficult. Attaching an economic value to improvements in health status and the avoidance of premature death is a real challenge and one that health economists have struggled with. A number of methods are used.

1. The Human Capital Approach: the projected future earnings of the individual are assumed to represent the economic value of life.
2. Socially Implied Valuations: the costs of public sector decisions that are designed to improve safety, such as road safety campaigns, imply the value of a human life.
3. Contingent Valuation: the value of healthcare programs are elicited from individuals who are asked to reveal the maximum they would be willing to pay to access some service or the minimum they would be willing to accept as a compensation for being denied access to a service.
4. Choice Experiments (or Conjoint Analysis): Individuals are asked to value a number of characteristics (or attributes) of the healthcare program such as waiting time, type of treatment, and type of staff who provided care. The valuations of these components can be used to identify the preference of valuation of a health program.

The "Contingent Valuation" and "Choice Experiment" methods are closest to how a market would find consumer valuations for goods and services, but these are still difficult to implement and have been criticized [20]. If the value of the benefits of healthcare can be accurately measured, then we are in a position to make some judgments about improving economic efficiency from reallocating resources in an economy, when markets will not do the job for us.

1.3   Conclusions

Making good choices over how scarce resources are allocated is important. Good choices provide greater benefit to society than bad choices. Efficient resource allocation will maximize benefits, and governments should try to make sure all individuals get a fair slice of the wealth generated. Competitive markets allocate resources efficiently. When markets go wrong, as they do for health care, then decisions about how to allocate resources have to be made manually. The best way to inform those decisions is to conduct an economic appraisal. Economic appraisal is an important part of the health economists' toolkit and one that infection-control practitioners can readily exploit in order to move scarce resources toward infection control, or reorganize how existing infection-control resources are used. The infection-control practitioner can use economics to improve efficiency in health care resource allocation.

Chapter 2
Health Economics

Preview

- The origins of health economics and the work health economists do are described.
- The parts of health economics that are useful to infection control professionals are highlighted.
- A particular interpretation of health economics that makes decision-making easier is described.

2.1 Origins and Content of Health Economics

Health economics has grown out of mainstream economics. Its birthday was in 1963, when Kenneth Arrow published a paper on how perfectly competitive markets and public sector agencies (i.e., nonmarket forces) shape the provision and distribution of health care services [21]. Arrows' seminal paper starts with a discussion of why perfectly competitive markets are useful for helping to organize an economic system and then suggests why healthcare is a special case that cannot be left to the market. He notes problems with information will cause market failure, misallocate resources, and so fail to promote economic efficiency in the healthcare sector. We discussed these and other problems toward the end of Chap. 1 and suggested that government (i.e., a nonmarket force) might step in to help things along. The manual process of economic appraisal of healthcare decisions can benefit the economy and society in place of poorly functioning competitive markets.

Health economics is the application of the discipline of economics to the topic of health and health care. An influential health economists, Alan Williams, became involved in this subdiscipline in the early 1970s. He subsequently wrote an expanded definition of health economics in 1987 [22] that included eight topics, which are summarized in Fig. 5. This is known as the plumbing diagram.

The plumbing diagram illustrates that health economics embraces a number of topics, that many of these are interrelated, and that health economists collaborate with other professions (e.g., doctors, politicians, and administrators) and academics (epidemiologists, statisticians, and bench scientists) [23].

N. Graves et al., *Economics and Preventing Healthcare Acquired Infection*,
DOI: 10.1007/978-0-387-72651-9_3, © Springer Science + Business Media, LLC 2009

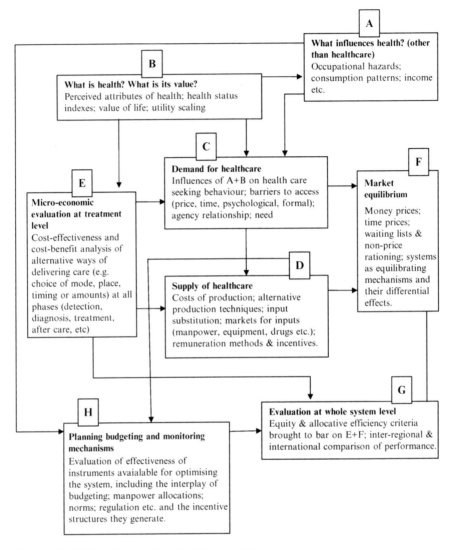

Fig. 5 Alan Williams' description of health economics

Box A is about factors other than healthcare interventions that influence health. Lifestyle choices like smoking and obesity are important determinants of health, as are education, poverty, ethnicity, and the physical environment. There are powerful arguments to be made about changing some of these factors – such as poverty and education – and so reducing the need for invasive and expensive health care services later in life. An example is using economics to inform policy on the regulation of tobacco advertising.

Box B is about measuring and valuing health outcomes. The RAND insurance experiment spawned the now widely used SF-36 health survey [24] that describes both physical and mental health and provides a quantitative score of health outcome across multiple dimensions of health. John Brazier and colleagues are health economists and devised a method for revaluing SF-36 data into a single health-related quality of life score between zero and 1, where zero is dead and 1 represents good health [25, 26]. The outcome measure might seem crude, but it is very useful for weighting the quality of additional years of life arising from some healthcare intervention. The "quality adjusted life year" (QALY) is the result and is used in health economics to describe the benefits of healthcare interventions in terms of how much health gain is produced by a decision to allocate resources to a certain health program. We describe and use the QALY later in this book. Infection control that prevents HAI will cause improved quality of life and may even reduce risk of death and so extend life.

Box C is about the demand for health care. This is related to the determinants of health and how health is measured and valued (i.e., Boxes A and B), since an individual's demand for health care depends on their state of health and how they value improvements in their state of health. The amount of health care any individual demands will also be governed by the price of health care, including nonfinancial costs over and above any professional fees and treatment costs, such as the loss of time it takes to access health care, and psychological factors such as fear of diagnosis and potential poor prognosis. Also, individuals have to use agents (e.g., doctors, health authorities, insurance companies) to demand healthcare, and these agency relationships add further complexity to the demand for healthcare. A nice case study is to imagine whether a patient newly admitted to hospital is able to adequately express their demand for infection control. It is unlikely they will be aware of the latest CDC guidelines or relevant research about risk and infection. For example, few patients would know there is increased risk of catheter colonization if a central line is inserted into the femoral vein rather than the subclavian [27]. The information deficit suffered by the patient illustrates the need for agents to act on their behalf when planning infection control services.

Box D is about the supply of healthcare and the resources used for the production of healthcare. Health economists might investigate why doctors earn 20 or 30 times more than highly skilled nurses in some health systems, explore how capital equipment, such as surgical robots, might substitute or complement human surgeons, and how drug companies might be coerced into lowering prices for life saving therapies. Infection control is one production process used in healthcare. Analyzing the resources used for infection control and how costs change with the scale and scope of infection-control activities falls under this heading.

Box E is about the microevaluation of healthcare programs, and this is another term for "economic appraisal" that was discussed at the end of Chap. 1 and the beginning of this chapter. The activity requires the assessment of the costs and the benefits of alternate ways of using scarce health care resources. It can be used to provide information that would have emerged from perfect markets, if these markets could be used to allocate scarce resource efficiently, which of course they cannot. The endpoint of an economic appraisal is some recommendation about whether a decision to use health care resources in one way over another is likely to improve efficiency within the healthcare sector. Given what we know about scarcity and the need to choose between competing uses of healthcare resources, microevaluation/economic appraisal is potentially powerful. If one healthcare intervention (e.g., MRSA screening) is shown to be better value for money than another (e.g., a surgical robot), and we know we cannot afford to do both, economic appraisal can be used to inform the decision about choosing between them. The microevaluation of healthcare programs is the most visible activity undertaken by those working with health economics because it can inform decision making directly. Many evaluation studies are undertaken each year, and they are often published in good quality medical journals such as JAMA and the New England Journal of Medicine. The methods are often used by noneconomist researchers. Many health care professionals such as doctors and nurses perform and publish economic evaluations. These microevaluations inform both the demand and supply sides of the health care industry. We spend a good amount of this book discussing how economic appraisal can be used for infection control.

Box F is about balancing the demand for health care with the supply of health care. One objective might be to find an efficient allocation of resources (remember economic efficiency from Chap. 1). The role of microevaluation (Box E) on the demand side (Box C) and the supply side (Box D) in finding an efficient outcome for the health care sector is consolidated by Box F.

Box G is about evaluating the entire health care system in terms of efficiency, equity, and cost containment. Crude international comparisons are often made on variables such as proportion of GDP devoted to health care production and life expectancy. For example, we know that US spends more than anyone else on health care but the Japanese live the longest.

Box H is about the assessment of policies that are used to regulate a health care system such as taxes and subsidies and other forms of intervention.

Health economics is a broad topic that can be complex, yet it is often intuitive and easy to interpret. To meet the aims of this book, we need to identify the parts of health economics that are most useful for the infection-control professional.

2.2   The Parts of Health Economics Most Useful for Infection-Control

An infection-control professional – like everybody else – will always face problems of scarcity, that is, wants always exceed means. You may want to implement any number of programs that will directly reduce risk of infection (i.e., use of antimicrobial catheters) or indirectly reduce risks of infection (i.e., staff awareness and education for hand washing), yet you do not have a sufficient budget or enough resources to do everything. You must choose what to do with your scarce resources (i.e., your staff and cash budgets). You should aim to be efficient and get the greatest benefit from your scarce resources. Exactly this question was the subject of a symposium at the Interscience Conference on Antimicrobial Agents and Chemotherapy meeting in San Francisco in 2006, and these were the topics of the symposium:

- Robert Sheretz spoke about "The Most Cost-Effective Way to Spend $100,000 in Infection Control: Investment in Personnel and Education"
- Craig Coopersmith spoke about "The Most Cost-Effective Way to Spend $100,000 in Infection Control: Investment in Infrastructure and Technology"
- Jacques Schrenzel spoke about "The Most Cost-Effective Way to Spend $100,000 in Infection Control: Investment in Microbiology"
- Sanjay Saint asked the question, "Is Infection Control Cost-Effective?"

In the absence of market mechanisms to allocate resources for infection control activities, economic appraisal can be used. You may wish to allocate more resources to infection-control and away from some other activity in the hospital such as outpatient services or cardiology services. You may want to reallocate your existing resources to some other use, such as away from staff education and toward prospective surveillance. You will improve your chances of achieving a reallocation if you make the economics clear for decision makers, and for this purpose, economic appraisal is useful.

There are many examples of how economic appraisal has been used to inform decisions about how to allocate scarce resources. One famous example of a micro-evaluation of a healthcare program (see Box E) was published in 1975 by Neuhauser and Lewicki [28]. They illustrated that testing a stool sample six-times to diagnose colorectal cancer would cost an extra $47 million per case detected. The first five tests were much cheaper per case detected. If a decision were made to allocate resources to six-times testing of stool samples then there would be a few, very grateful patients whose cancer was diagnosed early and cured. The relevant question is what else has been foregone from the millions of dollars allocated to the true positive diagnoses found from the sixth test? Think back to the discussion of opportunity costs in Chap. 1? It is likely that many more lives could have been saved by allocating resources to other competing activities such as expanding vaccination programs, funding drug and alcohol education in schools, and HIV prevention programs.

The economics of a proposal made by a group Duke University cell biologists is another interesting case [29]. They found the incidence of pressure ulcers among hospitalized patients had been reduced but not eliminated despite the use of air-fluidized beds and other specialty devices. They argued that in the future, high risk patients may be sent to space clinics to recuperate in zero gravity for extended periods. Although an appealing solution for a cell biologist, it makes little sense to an economist. We know space travel with existing technology is expensive (see Fig. 2 in Chap. 1), and so the opportunity costs of this decision would be enormous. The resources tied up by providing therapy in the Earth's orbit could be used more productively in other parts of the terrestrial health care system.

Economic appraisal is potentially useful in the healthcare sector as a method of promoting efficiency in resource allocation. To undertake an economic appraisal, we need to use techniques from some of the other boxes in Williams' plumbing diagram. For instance, we will need to know how to estimate the costs of HAIs and the costs of infection control programs. This will use Box D, which is about how healthcare is produced. We will also need to know how to measure and value health outcomes, this will use Box B. We also need to think about the microevaluation at treatment level, the subject of Box E. A number of other disciplines must be involved: clinical expertise is required and we will have to use some epidemiology and statistics. The process of economic appraisal is genuinely multidisciplinary. Although health economics is about more that just economic appraisal (Box E), for now we focus on these techniques. They are powerful and potentially useful for infection control professionals. We describe the different approaches to economic appraisal next.

2.3   Competing Approaches to Economic Appraisal

There are two broad schools of thought about economic appraisal in healthcare and these compete head to head. Competent users of economics should be aware of the differences. The distinctions are often glossed over in papers that discuss the application of economic evaluation for healthcare. First is the *welfarist* approach that only includes cost-benefit analysis (CBA). Second are *extra-welfarist* approaches that include cost-effectiveness analysis (CEA) and a special form of CEA, cost-utility analysis (CUA). One type of economic appraisal, cost-minimization analysis (CMA), is not useful for decision making in healthcare [30]. A failure to discriminate between welfarism and extra-welfarism could lead to mistakes in the choice of the method used, a failure to apply the method properly and a failure to correctly interpret and report findings. The different methods and the two schools of thought are summarized in Fig. 6.

The advocates for either approach measure the *costs* and *benefits* of competing healthcare interventions to make decisions that promote efficiency. However, despite the apparent similarities, irreconcilable differences exist.

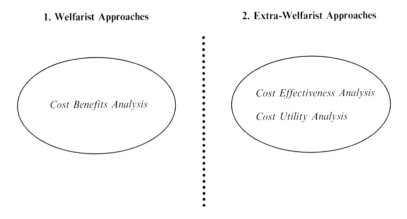

1. Welfarist Approaches   **2. Extra-Welfarist Approaches**

Cost Benefits Analysis

Cost Effectiveness Analysis

Cost Utility Analysis

Economists debate which approach is better.

Fig. 6 Welfaist and extra-welfarist approaches to economic appraisal

2.3.1   *Welfarism*

Welfarists believe that the benefits of a health care intervention should be valued by individual consumers in the same way that any other goods and services are valued. This implies that a consumer will choose the types of healthcare, alongside other goods and services that provide the maximum personal benefit. Individuals are thought to be the best judges of what makes them happy. Welfarists focus on human behavior. If a welfarist sat down on a Sunday evening and planned their weekly shop (i.e., their allocation of resources), it might read something like this:

Things I will buy this week (given scarce resources)

- Dozen Apples, five oranges, and two kiwi fruit
- Cheese balls (packet of 12)
- Dog food
- Calcium supplements to reduce bone loss and risk of fracture in the future
- New socks
- Diet and exercise program to mitigate risk of cardiovascular event
- Beastie Boys album
- Visit path lab for MRSA swab prior to visiting sick relative in ICU
- Cinema tickets
- Repair sole on work shoes

Things I will do without this week (given scarce resources)

- Olive oil (5 L)
- Have test for prostate cancer
- Replace the bald tire on the car
- Visit dentist

This way of thinking arises from the notion of competitive markets, the price mechanism, and the invisible hand, which were all discussed in Chap. 1. Welfarists assume people can find out what healthcare they want and are able to reveal their individual valuation of the benefits of healthcare relative to all other uses of scarce resources. The result is that they choose to consume just the right mix of goods and services to maximize their utility or happiness. We can summarize this argument by a review of the data in Table 3.

The cost of the items are presented in the second column, the dollar valuations of the benefits of consuming these items are presented in the third column and the net benefits, the benefit less the cost (or the profit consumers enjoy), in the fourth. We have sorted these items by the size of the net benefit, so those items consumers value highest are at the top of the list. To be efficient and so gain the most from our scarce resources, we maximize the sum of the net benefits. If our income is $250 per week, then we work down the list until all our income is allocated between the items. The $250 is exhausted after we have consumed items 1–10, as follows:

$$\$75 + \$25 + \$10 + \$50 + \$12 + \$10 + \$15 + \$10 + \$5 + \$38 = \$250$$

Net benefit is also maximized:

$$\$25 + \$10 + \$5 + \$5 + \$5 + \$3 + \$4 + \$4 + \$3 + \$3 = \$67.$$

Any reallocation of our resources to include items 11–14 will reduce the total of net benefits and so lead to a less efficient outcome. The reason is that the net benefit of items shaded in gray is less than the minimum net benefit of any of the items not shaded. You can confirm this by substituting any of items 11–14 for any items 1–10 (but remember you have only got $250 to play with). If we took number 2 (calcium + Vitamin D) and number 9 (Cheese balls) out of our list and replaced them with number 11 (Olive Oil), then we have still spent $250 but have reduced out net benefits to $56, and we have achieved less from the same resources. The efficient outcome is to buy items 1–10 and none of items 11–14.

We know that markets fail in health care and so the information summarized in Table 3, which would have arisen so easily in a perfectly competitive market, must be collected manually via economic appraisal. To use economic appraisal, we therefore need a method to identify the costs and benefits of all the available programs. Without this information, it is difficult to find an efficient allocation of scarce resources. Welfarists believe this information can be provided via one form of economic appraisal called cost-benefit analysis. Those who conduct cost-benefit analyses for healthcare decisions try to understand the consumer's preference (i.e., dollar valuation) for health care, just as would have been revealed in a competitive market for sneakers, food, or clothing. This preference is expressed by a dollar valuation of the benefits of healthcare (i.e., the third column in Table 3.). We made a comment in Chap. 1 that valuing the benefits of health care in dollar

Table 3 The cost, benefit and net benefit of possible consumption alternatives

Items that we have valuedw	Cost	Benefit[a]	Net benefit
1. New diet/exercise program to mitigate risk of cardiovascular event	$75	$100	$25
2. Begin a course of calcium + vitamin to reduce bone loss and risk of fracture	$25	$35	$10
3. Beastie Boys new album	$10	$15	$5
4. Visit path lab for MRSA swab prior to visiting sick relative in ICU	$50	$55	$5
5. Dog food	$12	$17	$5
6. New socks	$10	$16	$3
7. Cinema tickets	$15	$19	$4
8. Dozen apples, five oranges, and two kiwi fruit	$10	$14	$4
9. Cheese balls (packet of 12)	$5	$8	$3
10. Repair sole on work shoes	$38	$41	$3
11. Olive oil (5 L)	$30	$32	$2
12. Replace the bald tire on the car	$80	$82	$2
13. Visit dentist	$250	$251	$1
14. Have test for prostate cancer	$500	$501	$1

[a]Benefit is the personal utility gained by consumers and is expressed in terms of their willingness to pay for benefits, relative to all other alternatives

terms is difficult and briefly described the methods at the end of the chapter. Health economists tend to use "contingent valuation" and "choice experiments" to find monetary values for health care programs, but these methods are not widely used and have been criticized [20].

An alternative to welfarism is extra-welfarism, and those who believe this approach is best, advocate the use of two different types of economic appraisal for the purpose of allocating resources, cost-effectiveness, and cost-utility analyses.

2.3.2 Extra-Welfarism

Extra-welfarists debate the assumption that individual consumers of health care should aim to maximize their personal satisfaction, as they would if consuming sneakers, food, or clothing. Extra-welfarists believe resources should be allocated to pursue the social objectives set by the social decision maker. In a health care context, the primary objective of the social decision maker is to maximize the total health of the population. The difference between welfarism and extra-welfarism is that one believes in maximizing personal satisfaction (i.e., happiness or utility) and that this can be expressed in dollar terms, to allow cost-benefit analysis, and the other believes in maximizing health, with all its dimensions such length of life, pain, mobility, anxiety, usual activities, and ability to self-care. The idea of individual consumer sovereignty and the competitive market is down-played by the extra-welfarists. Extra-welfarism takes a paternalistic approach, tasking government, and other external groups to make recommendations about what healthcare people need, how it should be produced and who gets it. Decision making about how scarce resources are used is taken away from individuals and handed over to government or quasi-government agencies who try to maximize health from scarce resources. The justification is that the decision maker.

'occupies his position by virtue of a socially approved political process. He has been entrusted with the task of making choices on behalf of the general public, and this trust implies that he will formulate objectives for the society.' [31]

The tools of extra-welfarism are cost-effectiveness analysis and cost-utility analysis. The analyst will measure the costs of competing healthcare interventions in monetary units and measure the benefits in terms of changes to health outcomes, not dollar values. An analyst undertaking a cost-effectiveness analysis will characterize health benefits in natural units of health outcome such as life years gained, pain free days, or nosocomial infections prevented. A cost-utility analysis is a special type of cost-effectiveness analysis with health benefits measured by quality adjusted life years (QALYs). See Panel 2 for an introduction to QALYs. This measure of benefit is quite different from the monetary valuation sought by welfarists and allows decision makers to maximize *health* from scarce resources.

For the purposes of this book, we choose to be extra-welfarists and so think about maximizing health benefits as measured by QALYs.

2.4   Advantages and Disadvantages of Each Type of Economic Appraisal

The welfarist method of cost-benefit analysis is attractive because it is designed to measure what matters to individuals. It accounts for the preferences of individuals for health alongside all the other things they might consume with scarce resources such as cheese balls, dog food, and socks. Because of the compensation principle described in Chap. 1, where the winners from a decision do not actually have to compensate the

A QALY is derived by measuring the increased duration of life from an intervention and then adjusting the extra years by quality weights. These weights take values between zero (dead) and 1 (good health).

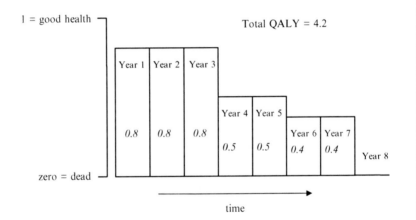

A patient without treatment faces certain death. Luckily for them, they receive a treatment that extends their life by seven years. Over the course of the seven years their quality of their life however will reduce.

during years 1 to 3 the value of the health state they occupy is 0.8
during years 4 and 5 the value is 0.5
during years 6 and 7 the value is 0.4

The total QALYs gained from the treatment is:
0.8 + 0.8 + 0.8 + 0.5 + 0.5 + 0.4 + 0.4 = 4.2 QALYs.

Had they been in good health, they would have enjoyed 7 QALYs.

The treatment generates health benefits valued at 4.2 QALYs.

Panel 2   The quality adjusted life year (QALY)

losers from a decision, a conceptually simple approach to maximizing benefits from scarce resources emerges. Cost-benefit analysis, however, requires individuals to attach a monetary valuation to benefits (see the data in Table 3) and this throws up two problems. One, the wealthy individuals are likely to be willing to pay more for health than the poor, so they may bias resource allocating decisions. Two, it is awkward to ask people to attach a monetary value to health outcomes and gathering the data summarized in Table 3 is a difficult process.

The extra-welfarist methods of CEA and CUA inform the narrower goal of maximizing health outcomes (e.g., measured by QALYs if CUA is chosen) from a fixed pot of resources, such as an annual budget for healthcare expenditures. The power is placed with a notional healthcare decision maker. This method is perceived to be easier to implement than CBA, but does suffer from some criticism, see Coast [32] and Donaldson [33]. A major criticism is that the "decision maker" may not be clearly identified. In reality, decisions are made at many levels and many time points by many different people each with varying objectives that may or may not represents societies objectives. Indeed the Coast paper, published in the BMJ [32] stimulated a lively debate between the welfarists and the extra-welfarists, which can be found on the BMJ Website for those who are interested in a good academic debate.

For the rest of this book, we are going to be extra-welfarists and aim to get the most health benefit from scarce resources to improve efficiency in the health care system. We believe this is closest to the situation faced by those who decide what to do with scarce healthcare resources that may be made available for infection control. It also sidesteps the need for difficult valuations of the benefits of infection control and because infection impacts on both quality and quantity of life, we think the QALY is a suitable outcome measure.

2.5   Conclusions

Health economics is multidisciplinary and broad in scope. The most useful part of health economics for infection control practitioners is economic appraisal. This allows the value for money of competing ways of using scarce health care resources to be assessed. There are two approaches to economic appraisal, welfarist and extra welfarist, and we discussed why we prefer the latter. We choose to describe the costs of health care programs in dollar terms and the benefits in either natural units of output, such as infections prevented or quality adjusted life years (QALYs). Cost-utility analyses – that use QALYs – is the more useful approach to economic appraisal as it allows many different types of health care programs to be compared using a common measure. Cost-utility analysis should be used to evaluate infection control programs.

Chapter 3
Economic Appraisal: A General Framework

Preview

- The general idea of economic appraisal is described.
- The results that emerge are reviewed.
- Advice is provided on how they should be interpreted for decision-making.

3.1 What an Economic Appraisal Looks Like

Economic appraisal is about measuring and valuing the costs and benefits that arise from a decision to change something. The theme for this book is how costs and health benefits change when changes are made to infection-control practices. We are interested in whether making changes to current infection control arrangements will improve efficiency or not. For this application we will be extra-welfarists and use cost-utility and cost-effectiveness analysis to address questions about efficiency.

For any economic appraisal we must define where to start the analysis. This provides a baseline or reference to which costs and health effects can be compared, after changes to infection-control practice have been implemented. The start point might be called "Existing Practice" and describes the current situation. Resources are then reallocated to a "New Program." Costs will change and health benefits will change as well. Decision-makers are interested in the change to both sets of economic outcomes. All possible changes to costs and health benefits are illustrated in Fig. 7 and this is called the cost-effectiveness plane.

The vertical axis is used to describe the *Costs* and the horizontal axis the *Health Benefits*. If a new program causes costs to decrease and health benefits to increase, then decision makers enjoy a "win, win" and they occupy a point in Quadrant II. Relative to existing practice costs are saved and health outcomes improve. Decision makers should always adopt programs like this: it would be unethical not to. A decision not to adopt a program that occupies Quadrant II causes unnecessary costs and simultaneously harms patients. Look at the position of Existing practice compared to any point in Quadrant II. The "New Program" can be thought of as

N. Graves et al., *Economics and Preventing Healthcare Acquired Infection*,
DOI: 10.1007/978-0-387-72651-9_4, © Springer Science + Business Media, LLC 2009

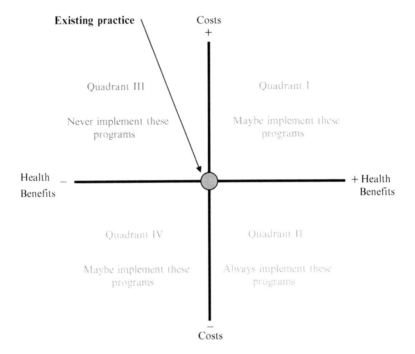

Fig. 7 The cost-effectiveness plane

"dominating" existing practice by both measures of cost and effect. It might be that infection-control programs are like this. Infections can be very expensive and preventing them can be quite cheap. Infection control may pay for itself (i.e., saves cost) and also generate health benefits because infections are avoided. If this were true then infection-control would occupy a point in the quadrant marked II.

If the "New Program" causes costs to rise and health benefits to decrease, then decision makers suffer a "lose, lose" because costs have been incurred while harming people; this is described by any point in Quadrant III. The decision to adopt an unsafe drug therapy is an example. If the therapy led to serious adverse events that decreased overall the quality or quantity of life for users, the health benefits would be reduced from a decision to use the drug. Costs would also have been increased as scarce resources would have been used up to develop and distribute the product. With this situation "Existing Practice" is said to dominate the "New Program" by cost and effect and these programs should never be implemented. Decision makers have a relatively easy time when the "New Program" ends up in either quadrants II or III and so either "dominates" or is "dominated."

Decision makers face a harder task when the "New Program" causes increased cost and health benefit, that is, the "New Program" lands on a point in Quadrant I, or, when the "New Program" saves cost and reduces health benefits and so lands on a point in Quadrant IV. Under these scenarios the decision maker must balance the change in cost with the change in benefit and then make a judgment about whether

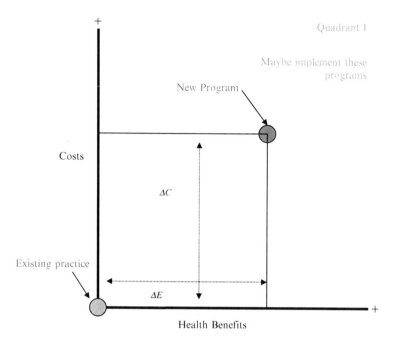

Fig. 8 Quadrant I of the cost-effectiveness plane with new program

the "New Program" is good value for money or not. A "New Program" that increases cost and health benefit is shown in Fig. 8; this is an enlargement of Quadrant I in Fig. 7. Programs that occupy a point in Quadrant IV are problematic because although they save costs they also reduce health benefits. It is likely to be difficult for policy makers to remove a program, once in place, if it can be shown to provide health benefits. More on this can be found in these two papers [34, 35].

The change in costs by adopting the "New Program" over "Existing Practice" is marked by ΔC on the vertical axis. The letter C stands for "cost" and the triangle is the uppercase of the fourth letter in the Greek alphabet and is called "Delta" and means the difference between two numbers. The two numbers are *costs at "Existing Practice"* and *costs after the "New Program" has been implemented*. The change in cost or "Delta cost" or ΔC is summarized like this

$$\Delta C = C(\text{NP}) - C(\text{EP}).$$

If the costs of existing practice (EP) were \$5,000 and the costs of the "New Program" (NP) were \$7,500, then "delta cost" or ΔC would be \$7,500 minus \$5,000 and this equals \$2,500.

Changes to health benefits are assessed the same way. Delta effect or ΔE is summarized like this

$$\Delta E = E(\text{EP}) - E(\text{NP}).$$

If the number of infections prevented with existing practice (EP) was 50 and the number of infections prevented with the "New Program" (NP) was 100, then "delta effect" or ΔE would be 50 minus 100 and this equals 50 less infections.

These two pieces of information can be used by decision makers to assess whether the intervention represents good value for money. The cost per unit of health benefit obtained (i.e., cost per infection prevented) can be calculated by dividing the change in costs ΔC by the change in health benefits ΔE which is $2,500 divided by 50 and this equals $50 per infection avoided. This is summarized in this complicated looking – but easy – formula below:

$$\frac{C(EP)-C(NP)}{E(EP)-E(NP)} = \frac{\Delta C}{\Delta E} = \frac{\$7,500-\$5,000}{100-50} = \frac{\$2,500}{50} = \$50/\text{HAI avoided.}$$

If the "New Program" is adopted then $50 is paid for each infection prevented. The slope of the line that joins "Existing Practice" to the "New Program" drawn in Fig. 9 summarizes an increase of $50 on the vertical axis for an increase of one infection avoided on the horizontal axis.

If more accurate data are collected and the true health benefits of the "New Program" are found to be only be 70 infections avoided, marked by point marked "A," then the gradient on the line is steeper and the cost per infection prevented is increased. This is shown by substituting 70 for 100 in this equation

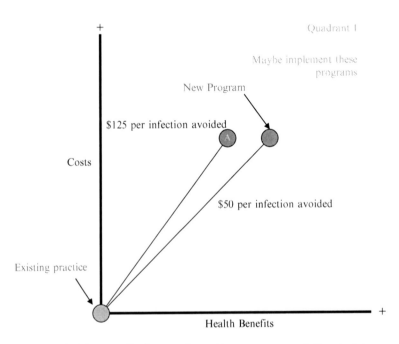

Fig. 9 Quadrant I of the cost-effectiveness plane with new program and alternate data

$$\frac{C(\mathrm{EP})-C(\mathrm{NP})}{E(\mathrm{EP})-E(\mathrm{NP})}=\frac{\Delta C}{\Delta E}=\frac{\$7,500-\$5,000}{70-50}=\frac{\$2,500}{20}=\$125\,/\,\mathrm{HAI\,avoided.}$$

In this case, decision makers pay $125 per one infection avoided. With the axes this way round, the shallower the gradient on the lines the lower the cost per infection avoided. The values of $50 and $125 per infection avoided are called "Incremental Cost-Effectiveness Ratios" (ICER). This term will be used throughout this book.

For this example ICERs have been calculated using dollar costs and the natural units of "infections avoided" and so this is a cost-effectiveness analysis. ICERs can also be calculated using QALYs as the measure of health gain and this would be a cost-utility analysis. We move on to cost-utility analysis in the next section, extend the example to consider more than one program and learn about the importance of thinking incrementally.

3.2   Incremental Analysis

Decisions based on economic appraisal must be considered in terms of incremental changes. This is particularly relevant when more than one infection control program is under consideration. Infection control professionals will often have to decide whether to remain with "Existing Practice" or choose one of many alternate programs. There are many ways of reducing risk of infection and our task is to choose the programs that are efficient. Some hypothetical data are included in Table 4 and Fig. 10 that describe the cost outcomes and health benefits (measured in QALYs) of "Existing Practice" and four competing infection control programs.

As before, the start of the analysis is "Existing Practice" which describes existing infection control arrangements. Decision makers face four further options. Program A can be discarded immediately because it is dominated by both cost and effect, that is, it causes higher costs and lower health benefits than Existing Practice and Programs B or D. Program B is superior to Program A because it is not dominated by any other program, however, the cost per unit of health benefit obtained (i.e., the ICER) is higher than for Program D.

Confirm this by examining the gradient of the line between "Existing Practice" and "Program B" and between "Existing Practice" and "Program D". The gradient is shallower for "Program D" and so the ICER is lower which means the cost per

Table 4   The cost and QALY outcomes

	Costs	QALYs
Existing Practice	$20,000	10
Program A	$210,000	2
Program B	$80,000	20
Program C	$300,000	175
Program D	$145,000	150

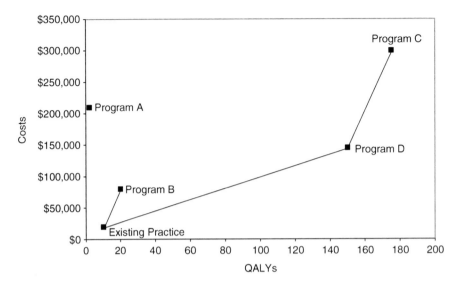

Fig. 10 The cost and QALY outcomes of five competing decisions

unit of health benefit is cheaper making "Program D" efficient (i.e., cost-effective) compared to Program B. If there was insufficient funding available to pursue "Program D" then "Program B" would still be discarded. Rather than choosing B over D, it would be better (i.e., more efficient) to choose some blend of "Existing Practice" and "Program D." This implies that some proportion of the population would receive "Program D" and the remainder would receive "Existing Practice." If we want to invest more scarce resources into infection control beyond those required for "Program D," then the only alternative is Program C.

The decision can be boiled down to choosing between "Existing Practice," Program D, and "Program C." These are all potentially efficient decisions, with Programs A and B representing inefficient decisions which are discarded. Incremental analysis now becomes critical. When choosing between the three potentially efficient decisions it is the change to costs and health benefits that must be analyzed. The data in Table 4 illustrate the incremental changes to costs and health benefits between the three potentially efficient programs.

A decision to implement Program D must be compared to Existing Practice and we see a change in costs (i.e., ΔC) of $125,000 and a change in QALYs of 140 (i.e., ΔE). The ratio of these two numbers is $893 (i.e., $125,000/140) and this is the incremental cost-effectiveness ratio for Program D. This is the correct number for decision making. It follows that the ICER for Program C is the ratio of the change in costs and change in QALYs as compared to Program D and this is $155,000 divided by 25 and this is $6,200 per QALY gained. Again this is the correct number for decision making. So we can summarize the analysis with these logical statements:

- Existing Practice and Programs B, D, and C are all better than Program A
- Existing Practice, Program D, and Program C are all potentially efficient

- A decision to choose Program C implies we are willing to pay $893 per QALY
- A decision to choose Program D implies we are willing to pay $6200 per QALY

The final step in choosing between Existing practice, Program C, and Program D requires us to make a normative judgment (i.e., a judgment on the value of something) about whether $893 or $6,200 represent good value for money as compared to alternative uses of scarce resources. This will depend on the maximum willingness to pay for health benefits (QALYs) by decision-makers. This maximum willingness to pay is called a ceiling ratio. If the relevant ceiling ratio was $8,000 per QALY then Program C would be implemented, if, however, it was $1,000 then Program C would be rejected and Program D would be selected. Finding appropriate values for ceiling ratios is considered in Sect. 3.3. This is resource allocation in practice and is grounded in the notion of efficiency. The process of economic appraisal, in the absence of a competitive market, is providing information about what should be done and how it should be done. Economics is concerned with answering these questions.

Often a gross error is made analyzing these types of data and the error appears in published papers. The problem is that "average" and not "incremental changes" are calculated. Average cost-effectiveness ratios assume each program is compared to…nothing at all. Look at the data in Table 5.

The interpretation of these numbers, with the average ratios in column four, is that we currently have no infection-control at all, and this is unlikely, there is normally basic infection-control in hospitals. Furthermore we assume that each intervention exists in isolation and so there is no point in making comparisons between them, again this is not a sensible way to analyze the information for decision making. We draw the average ratio for each option in Fig. 11.

The numbers that emerge from the average analysis contradict the ICERs presented in Table 5 and they will mislead decision makers. They suggest, for example, the cost per QALY of Program C is $1,714 when the ICER, the correct estimate for decision making, is actually $6,200. Torgerson and Spencer [36] make a clear distinction between incremental and average analyses and if you would like to rerun this point you might read their paper.

Table 5 The cost and QALY outcomes with misleading average ratios

	Costs	QALYs	Average ratios (costs/QALYs)
Existing Practice	$20,000	5	$4,000
Program A	$210,000	14	$15,000
Program B	$80,000	20	$4,000
Program C	$300,000	175	$1,714
Program D	$145,000	150	$967

An easy way to think about the incremental changes and the decision-making is to imagine that you have made a decision to buy a new car. The new car will cost $40,000 and that is a sufficient rate of return as compared to alternative ways of using your scarce resources. Now think about optional extras: alloy wheels are $2,000, air conditioning is $500 and the matching luggage set is $5,000. The decision about the optional extras will involve you comparing the change in costs (ΔC) with

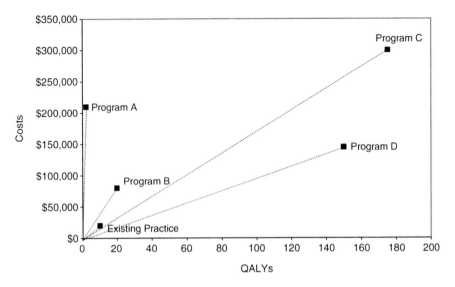

Fig. 11 Average cost-effectiveness ratios for five decisions: these are misleading

the change in benefits (ΔE) for each optional extra. It might be you judge the ratio of cost to return sufficient to justify the wheels and air conditioning but the ratio of cost to return for the luggage is an inefficient use of resources. You have been thinking incrementally and this is how things are done for economic analyses.

Whether we think the extra $893 per QALY from program D or $6,200 per QALY from Program C represents good value for money depends on the other ways of using the money in the healthcare sector and the total amount of money available. If other interventions provide cheaper QALYs (i.e., better value for money), then they might be chosen first. Decision makers often choose a maximum threshold willingness to pay for QALYs, to allow them to make decisions. This "ceiling ratio" is the topic for the next section.

3.3   Ceiling Ratios and Choosing Healthcare Programs

Finding an appropriate ceiling ratio or maximum willingness to pay for health benefits is easy in theory but in practice has proved difficult. The theory states that all health programs competing for the scarce pot of resources are ranked by their ICER. Those that produce the best ICERs, the best value for money, are selected first and decision makers work their way down the list until the available resources are exhausted. Health Programs that fall below the line and so have an ICER that is too expensive are not provided. This mechanism will maximize health benefits for a given budget and this is efficient. Milton Weinstein uses a book chapter to explain these arguments in detail [37].

A group of researchers at the Health Economics Research Centre at Oxford University set up a database of all cost-effectiveness studies published between 1997 and 2003 that reported cost per QALY gained and ranked them based on value for money: they found 199 separate studies. At the bargain basement end of the list was the use of Calcium + vitamin D compared to no treatment for women aged 70 with established osteoporosis [38]. This was found to save costs and generate health benefits. This was a "win, win" for decision makers and would land in Quadrant II of the cost-effectiveness plane. The use of cognitive behavioral therapy compared to treatment as usual for depression and anxiety among patients having experienced at least one episode of major unipolar depression was found to cost £2,111 per QALY [39]. Decision makers should adopt this program as it represents excellent value for money. The use of Docetaxel over Vinorelbine to treat advanced breast cancer among women requiring chemotherapeutic treatment for anthracycline-resistant advanced cancer is not such a clear cut decision because each QALY costs £18,591 [40]. There may be other ways of using resources that are more efficient (i.e., a lower cost per QALY gained). Decision makers should run a mile from using silicone adjustable gastric banding instead of gastric bypass for morbid obesity among patients diagnosed as morbidly obese (BMI > 40) with serious comorbid disease, in whom previous nonsurgical interventions failed. The cost per QALY for this decision was £303,566 [41]. There are definitely better ways of spending money for health care than making this decision. Primary prevention of diabetes, for example, is likely to get more QALYs per dollar spent.

An infection-control professional should be interested in finding out where various infection-control programs rank on such a list. Generating this type of list for an entire health system requires a huge volume of research and data to be synthesized. A group from the Harvard Center for Risk Analysis did make an attempt to rank healthcare interventions by ICER. They found 228 cost-utility analyses that reported ICERs for 647 health programs. Ten per cent of these were located in Quadrant II on the cost-effectiveness plane. Sixty four were dominated by other interventions, that is, there were cheaper and most effective alternative programs available. They found that 69% of the programs had ICERs of $50,000 or less and 78% had ICERS of $78,000 or less. In practice, choosing the appropriate cut off for programs, or finding a ceiling ratio for real world decision-making is difficult.

Alan Garber and Charles Phelps wrote a paper about economic appraisal in healthcare [42] arguing

> "most practitioners of CE analysis (economic appraisal) discard interventions with CE values (i.e., ICERs) at the top range ......, and conclude that interventions in the realm of $50,000 (or so) per QALY are "OK" but that more expensive technologies become more and more "out of bounds"; the $50,000 criterion is arbitrary and owes more to being a round number than to a well-formulated justification for a specific dollar value."

They went on to highlight an argument made by Phelps and Mushlin [43] some years earlier that stated

> "this leaves unresolved, or course, why interventions with relatively low marginal CE ratios (ICERs) are not expanded in scope at the expense of more costly interventions, a shift of medical resources that would surely increase health absolutely"

Infection-control is quite cheap and may even be cost saving, and will definitely deliver health benefits (QALYs). Even if infection control is not cost saving it might be that many programs have good (i.e., low) ICERs and so represents the type of program Phelps and Mushlin describe.

The cost per QALY and ICER arguments reviewed in this chapter are potentially powerful tools for infection-control professionals who wish to reallocate resources within current infection-control or increase the gross level of resources available at the expense of other areas of healthcare spending. Of course this will incur an opportunity cost elsewhere in the system, but if any reallocation can be shown to improve efficiency then a rational case for adoption exists.

One criticism of this approach to reallocating resources is that the studies from which ICERs emerge vary in quality and use inconsistent methods, assumptions, data, and analytic techniques. Much has been written about how to perform good quality economic appraisal [44–46]. We review some issues relevant to conducting economic appraisal in Chap. 4.

3.4 Conclusions

Economic appraisal is a summary of how costs and health benefits change with a decision to reallocate resources toward a new healthcare program. It is important to think about incremental changes and not just average changes. If costs fall and health benefits increase the decision is easy, but most of the time costs and health benefits increase together. When this happens, decision-makers need to choose a maximum willingness to pay for health benefits. This will help them discriminate between programs that are likely to improve efficiency and those that are not.

Chapter 4
Economic Appraisal: The Nuts and Bolts

Preview

- A method for economic appraisal is described.
- The different steps in the process are reviewed.
- Some aspects of a good quality study are discussed.

4.1   Using a Clinical Trial vs. a Modeling Study

Published economic appraisals fall into two groups: economic appraisal alongside clinical trials and economic appraisal by modeling study.

4.1.1   Economic Appraisal Alongside Clinical Trials

Economic appraisals are often conducted alongside clinical trials, randomized or not. Some consider economic appraisal alongside a randomized controlled trial to be the gold standard. This comes from an epidemiological view that randomizing patients between a control and intervention is likely to produce the best evidence about the cost-effectiveness of a health care program. This argument falters when we consider the complexity of an economic appraisal. To conduct a high quality appraisal, the analyst will need estimates of how effective a health program might be in preventing or curing disease, and these data should indeed be generated from an RCT. However, information is also required on other parameters that will affect costs and benefits. These might include understanding the risk of other events some of which are unlikely to occur with the time period of the trial. Examples are the use of health services in the future or long-term health outcomes, including mortality. Bacterial endocarditis may cause chronic and long-term health problems that persist beyond the end of a clinical trial designed to measure the effectiveness of a program that reduces the risk of blood stream infection. These health problems may

N. Graves et al., *Economics and Preventing Healthcare Acquired Infection*,
DOI: 10.1007/978-0-387-72651-9_5, © Springer Science + Business Media, LLC 2009

be very costly to treat and may reduce the quality and quantity of life for the patients affected. There may also be rare events among the entire population of patients that are unlikely to be observed during a clinical trial that includes a sample of patients. Crnich and Maki [47] make this point by suggesting that an RCT would need between 8,000 and 17,000 patients in each arm to show whether an antimicrobial coated central venous catheter reduced patient mortality. A decision maker is likely to require data on the performance of multiple competing health programs if they are to make a good decision that considers the costs and benefits of all relevant alternatives. It is unlikely that one RCT could be designed to accommodate more than two or three competing treatments, otherwise it would be too expensive, time consuming, and may cause ethical concerns. The evidence for some of the programs relevant to the decision maker may already be available, and it would be wasteful to reproduce this evidence in a new clinical trial. There are many reasons why an RCT might not be the best way to generate cost-effectiveness data for decision making. In contrast to economic appraisal conducted alongside clinical trials are model-based evaluations.

4.1.2   Economic Appraisal by Modeling Study

Those who choose to conduct an economic appraisal by using a modeling study synthesize evidence from a range of sources and combine all the information in a coherent decision-analytic process. The advantages of model-based appraisals is that events can be included that are not observed within a clinical trial (i.e., long-term cost and mortality outcomes or rare events) and programs that have not or cannot be directly compared in a clinical trial can be evaluated side by side in one coherent framework. This allows the consideration of all relevant competing infection-control interventions and not just a single novel strategy when compared with existing practice. Also, model-based appraisals are more generalizable and can be used to evaluate the cost-effectiveness of an intervention in a particular patient group, or in a "real-life" context often not represented by single clinical trials.

A good example of the modeling approach is a study published by Lindsay Frazier in JAMA [48] on the economics of choosing between different health programs for population-based colorectal cancer screening. Twenty one competing screening programs were compared with a do nothing alternative with long-term cost and mortality outcomes included in the estimation of costs and benefits. It would have been impossible to conduct this study as a prospective clinical trial. The results of their analyses are presented in Fig. 12, on the cost-effectiveness plane. They marked costs on the horizontal axis and benefits on the vertical axis and so all strategies that are dominated (i.e., more costly and less effective) are south-east of the efficient strategies. The axes are the opposite way round to all the examples presented so far. All efficient strategies are joined by the solid line.

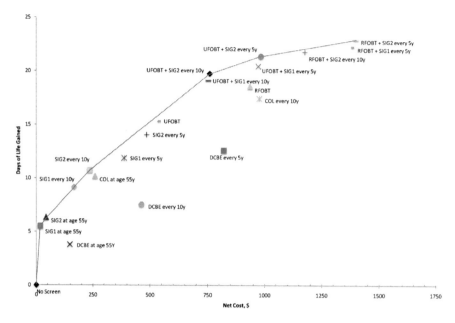

Fig. 12 The costs and health benefits of competing strategies for colorectal cancer screening

These results can be interpreted in exactly the same way as we have done before. The efficient strategies (and ICERs) are:

Sig 1 at age 55 yrs. = ICER of $1200 per LYG
Sig 2 at age 55 yrs. = ICER of $11,000 per LYG
Sig 1 every 10 yrs. = ICER of $15,800 per LYG
Sig 2 every 10 yrs. = ICER of $16,100 per LYG
UFOBT + SIG2 every 10 yrs. = ICER of $21,200 per LYG
UFOBT + SIG2 every 5 yrs. = ICER of $51,200 per LYG
RFOBT + SIG2 every 5 yrs. = ICER of $92,900 per LYG

Notes:

LYG = Life Year Gained
Sig 1 = sigmoidoscopy followed by colonoscopy if high risk poly diagnosed
Sig 2 = sigmoidoscopy followed by colonoscopy if high or low risk poly
        diagnosed
UFOBT = unrehydrated faecal occult blood test
RFOBT = rehydrated faecal occult blood test

An interpretation of these findings are that these strategies listed on the previous page are productively efficient, that is they are the cheapest way of obtaining health benefits (we are *"doing things right"*) and the other strategies, that do not touch the line in Fig. 12, are not productively efficient. The next question of choosing to provide the correct goods and services addresses questions of allocative efficiency or, *"doing the right things."* This depends on how much we are prepared to pay for a unit of health benefit (you might like to review the material in Chap. 1 on efficiency to remind yourself of the difference between productive and allocative efficiency). If society is willing to pay $20,000 per life year gained, then we choose Sig2 every 10 years. The next most effective program, UFOBT + SIG2 every 10 yrs, is too costly. It is inefficient as we believe these scarce resources can be used in a better way elsewhere in the economy. If, however, decision-makers are willing to pay $51,201 per LYG, then we choose the more effective UFOBT + SIG2 every 5 years.

4.2   Building a Model

Decision analytic models have been viewed with suspicion by some parts of the medical and academic community, in part due to the opaque nature of the methods and lack of clarity in how they were reported. The editors of the New England Journal of Medicine suggested the methods were "discretionary" [49], and argued this research tool could be misused by those who might profit from the adoption of a particular technology or intervention. There are now guidelines for how models should be developed and evaluated [46, 50, 51], and they must survive peer review if they are to be published in scientific journals. Regulatory agencies such as the National Institute for Clinical Excellence in the UK send models for detailed dissection and review by independent academics. Modeling studies are now published regularly in the best medical journals, see for example Frazier et al. [12] in JAMA, Golan et al. [13] in the Annals of Internal Medicine, Ades et al. [14] in the BMJ and Mann et al. [15] in the New England Journal of Medicine. Models are a vehicle for bringing together many different types of information that will help us decide whether resources should be put into a program or not.

Decision analytic models should be as simple as possible, to reduce the question in hand to its essentials, and they should be transparent, such that other investigators can build the model and test it with new data for a different setting or patient group. To develop a high quality decision model, we suggest a collaborative approach to include health care professionals with the relevant clinical experience, epidemiologists, statisticians, and either health economists or decision modellers. There are five objectives for a good decision model proposed by one of the leading contributors to economic appraisal in health care, Michael Drummond (p. 278 in [50]). We review the objectives next.

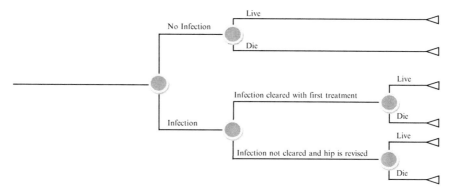

Fig. 13 The possible outcomes for patients at risk of infection following hip replacement

4.2.1   Objective One: Define the Structure of the Model

A structure that reflects the possible prognoses of the patients should be drawn. For the sake of example, we draw the possible outcomes for patients at risk of infection following total hip replacement in Fig. 13.

In this model, patients either develop an infection or they do not. If they develop an infection, they receive treatment to which they might respond. If they respond the infection is cleared. If they do not, then the primary prosthesis is removed and the infection is treated aggressively for 3–6 months to ensure eradication of the organism. Once confirmed, the hip revision procedure is performed with antibiotic cover and the revision prosthesis inserted. The end point for patients, no matter which of these clinical pathways they find themselves on, is that they will either live or die. This model considers the entire lifetime of patients and because hips are replaced at around 70 years of life, the model will have to describe events that project 10–20 years into the future.

This simple structure will be used to evaluate the cost-effectiveness of a novel infection-control program, the additional use of antibiotic cement during hip replacement, and compare this to an existing infection-control alternative, which is not to use the antibiotic cement. The cost and health benefit outcomes for those who receive the novel program are compared with those who do not. The decision model must reflect both alternatives, and this is illustrated in Fig. 14. Note that the top and bottom halves have an identical structure.

The square at the left side of the model is called a decision node. This is where a choice is made between the two alternatives, after careful consideration of the events that occur to the right. There are circles, which we call "probabilities," and triangles, which we call "payoffs," also included in the model structure.

Probabilities: The circles are called probability or chance nodes and represent events that will occur with some probability or chance. For example, a patient in the "Existing Program" may or may not get an infection and this probability is summarized

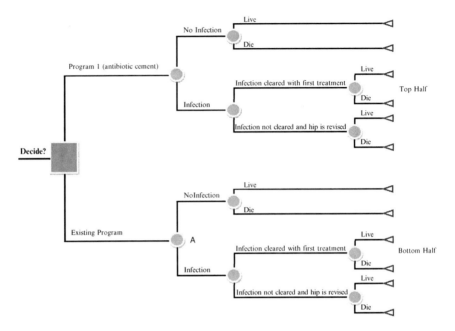

Fig. 14 A choice between two competing infection control alternatives (no data)

by the circle marked with an A in Fig. 14. It is important that the probabilities for each chance node add up to 1. If the probability a patient gets an infection at point A is 0.1, then the probability they do not is 1 minus 0.1 and this equals 0.9. A model will need data for every probability node that describe the chance of the event happening.

Payoffs: The triangles represent the final outcomes for patients that have traveled down any particular path. A patient in Program 1 without infection who lives will have different outcomes to a patient in Program 1, who gets an infection, has their hip revised, and then dies. For economic appraisal, the cost outcomes and the health benefit outcomes are estimated. Costs are measured by the money valuations of the resources used up for the patient that follows a given path to a triangle. The health benefits can be measured in common natural units, such as number of infections for traditional CEA, or health benefits can be expressed as QALYs for a CUA. Once the structure has been defined, we need data to describe the probabilities of all the chance events happening (circles) and then values for the various final outcomes (triangles).

4.2.2 Objective Two: Find the Evidence Required to Make the Decision

Evidence for the probabilities: The chance of the events to the right of the square decision node happening will be based on existing evidence, either from the published literature or from routine data. For example, surveillance data can be used to identify

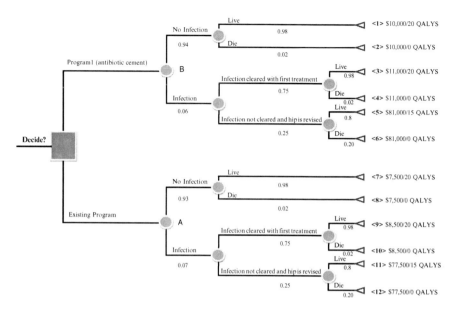

Fig. 15 A choice between two competing infection control alternatives (data included)

the risk of infection with existing infection-control programs. If the probability of infection under the existing program is 7%, then the probability of no infection is 100% less 7% = 93%. This evidence is marked on the model illustrated in Fig. 15 (see A in Fig. 15). This chance node sums to 1 (0.93 + 0.07).

Note the chance of infection is lower (only 6%) with the novel infection-control program (see B in Fig. 15). The novel program is effective and reduces risk of infection. The information on effectiveness may have been synthesized from a single RCT or from a metaanalysis of many studies. The probability that people will die (2%) is the same for the no infection pathways and the pathway for patients who have the infection cleared with the first treatment. The evidence for this can be obtained from mortality statistics, which are collected routinely and widely available for health care systems. The problematic patients who do not respond to treatment face a revision of the hip, and because this is a risky procedure, they face a greater chance of dying (20%). The evidence for this can be accessed from orthopedic registers of outcomes, which are collected by surgeons.

Evidence for the payoffs: Evidence is also needed to describe the cost and benefit consequences of all pathways. These are summarized at the triangles, which are called terminal nodes. Each triangle summarizes the cost and QALY outcomes for the pathway that traces right to left, back to the square decision node. You can see the first triangle marked <1> indicates the costs and QALYs of the survivors, who do not get an infection and were treated under the novel infection-control program. They incurred costs of $10,000 and enjoyed 20 quality adjusted life years (QALYs) after discharge from hospital. In contrast, the patients who end up at <6> (i.e., they died following a revision of the hip after receiving the novel infection-control program) incurred costs of $81,000 and contribute 0 quality adjusted life years (QALYs). At this stage, we refrain from discussing how to measure the costs of infection and the costs of infection control, instead these issues are dealt with in Chaps. 6 and 7, respectively. We also refrain from discussing how to measure QALYs, this is covered in Chap. 8. For now just accept the data reported for <1> to <12> in Fig. 15 are accurate and describe the cost and QALY outcomes arising from each path in the tree.

4.2.3   Objective Three: Evaluate the Model that has been Designed

The process of model evaluation will translate the evidence selected into estimates of the cost and benefit of the program. These can be used to inform decision-making. The model has been built using an appropriate structure, and the evidence required to make the decision has been identified and included. The next step is to calculate or evaluate the model. This process is based on the expected outcomes of each competing decision at the decision node. The existing infection-control program and the novel program will generate expected costs and expected benefits. By starting at the terminal nodes (triangles) and then moving right to left, toward the square decision node, combining the outcome with the probability of that outcome, the expected value of costs and benefits at the square decision node are calculated. The process is illustrated with a simple example, illustrated in Panel 3, and then the data included in the example drawn in Fig. 15 are evaluated.

Now the method has been shown, we return to the example with the data drawn in Fig. 15. The cost and benefit outcomes are evaluated using exactly the same way and the results illustrated in Fig. 16. You might want to check them yourself. The results of this decision analytic model are summarized in Table 6.

The change to cost, ΔC, is $2,332.5 and the change to benefits ΔE is 0.019 QALYs, this is an ICER of $122,763.16 per QALY. These data, therefore, occupy a point in Quadrant I of the cost-effectiveness plane in Fig. 17.

It is unlikely that this program would be adopted at $122,763.16 per QALY as this is likely to exceed the decision makers maximum willingness to pay for health benefits. There may be other, more cost-effective, ways of buying QALYs with infection control. Consider four additional programs that compete directly with the antibiotic cement (Program 1) and the existing program. We extend the model to include these and present the results in Table 7. For clarity, the programs are listed in order of increasing cost.

The cost and benefit outcomes as well as the incremental changes to cost and benefits are described, and these data are plotted in Fig. 18.

Program 1 is dominated by Program 4, which is better value for money. The same applies to Programs 2 and 3. Only the Existing Program, Program 4 and Program 5 are potentially efficient. If $35,273.28 per QALY that arises from Program 4 is below the threshold ceiling ratio for efficient decision making,

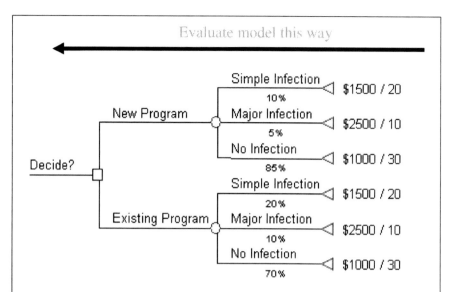

The expected cost of the 'New Program' is calculated by the sum of the actual costs of each outcome multiplied by the probability of that outcome.

- ✓ The expected cost is ($1500*10% = $150) + ($2500*5% = $125) + ($1000*85% = $850) = $150 + $125 + $850 = $1,125.
- ✓ The expected benefit is (20*10% = 2) + (10*5% = 0.5) + (30*85% = 25.5) = 2 + 0.5 + 25.5 = 28 QALYs.

The expected cost of the 'Existing Program' is calculated in the same way.

- ✓ The expected cost of the 'Existing Program' is ($1500*20% = $300) + ($2500*10% = $250) + ($1000*70% = $700) = $300 + $250 + $700 = $1250.
- ✓ The expected benefit is (20*20% = 4) + (10*10% = 1) + (30*70% = 21) = 4 + 1 + 21 = 26 QALYs.

The New Program provides 28 QALYs at a cost outcome of $1,125 vs. the Existing Program that provides 26 QALYs at a cost of $1,250.

Panel 3 An illustration of how to evaluate a decision model

then it should be chosen, and if this is too high then we should remain with the Existing Program. It is unlikely that decision makers would choose to spend the extra $7,720 for the additional 0.0076 QALYs implied by program 5; this means we spend $1,015,789.47 per QALY and is not a good use of scarce resources.

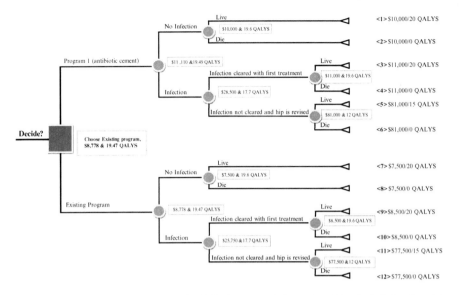

Fig. 16 A choice between two competing infection control alternatives (data included and model evaluated)

Table 6 Costs and QALYs of existing vs. novel infection control

	Costs	ΔC	QALYs	ΔE
Existing Infection-control Program	$8,778		19.47	
Novel Infection-control Program (Program 1)	$11,110	$2,332,5	19.49	0.019

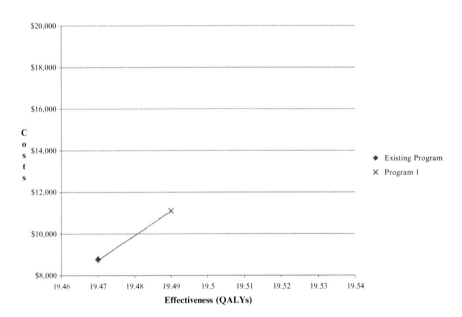

Fig. 17 Costs and QALYs of existing vs. novel infection control

Table 7 Costs and QALYs of existing vs. five novel infection control programs

Strategy	Cost	Incr cost (ΔC)	Eff	Incr eff (ΔE)	Incr C/E (ICER)
Existing Program	$8,777.5		19.47 QALY		
Program 4	$10,520	$1,742.5	19.52 QALY	0.0494 QALY	$35,273.28
Program 2	$11,017	$497	19.50 QALY	−0.0209 QALY	(Dominated)
Program 1	$11,110	$590	19.49 QALY	−0.0304 QALY	(Dominated)
Program 3	$14,376.5	$3,856.5	19.47 QALY	−0.0475 QALY	(Dominated)
Program 5	$18,240	$7,720	19.52 QALY	0.0076 QALY	$1,015,789.47

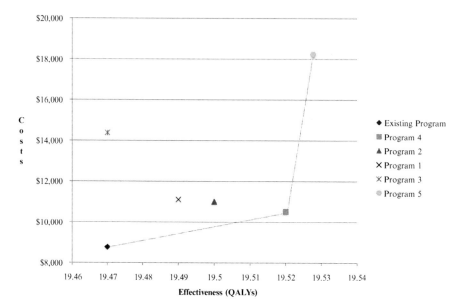

Fig. 18 Costs and QALYs of existing vs. five novel infection control programs – graphed

4.2.4   Objective Four: Account for Heterogeneity and Uncertainty

The results derived from an evaluation represent the best estimate of the cost-effectiveness of our competing interventions. However, it is important to recognize that decision modeling, just like decision making, is influenced by uncertainties in the information available. Briggs [52] identifies key sources of uncertainties, the first being generalizability of the results. Generalizability is about the contexts within which the results of a model may be valid. It requires consideration of heterogeneity in clinical contexts and patient groups. Heterogeneity arises naturally, for instance assumptions made about mortality and the effectiveness of the infection-control programs may be quite different for different age groups and data

can be collected to reflect this. Decision analytic models can, therefore, be cus-
tomized and adapted to describe different populations and even different settings
such as tertiary referral hospitals or country/district hospitals, which may have
different underlying rates of HAI and different types of patient. Adept modelers
will be able to evaluate heterogeneous groups in one modeling framework. An
example is an evaluation of Protein C for treatment of severe sepsis, which was
shown to be cost-effective for patients with an APACHE score ³25 but not for
patients with an APACHE score <25 [53].

Other sources of uncertainty arise from the structure of the evaluation and the
methods used in the evaluation. Many assumptions and decisions are made in struc-
turing and constructing the model. If important events are omitted or if the order of
events is not appropriate then some uncertainty will be carried forward to the
conclusions. Similarly the choice of timeframe or perspective to be used for the
evaluation will influence the results. These types of uncertainty are best considered
by using standard economic approaches to construct the model and conducting a
small number of alternate analyses, which look at the impact that changes to key
assumptions in the model have on results.

The final type of uncertainty arises from the data used to describe the parameters
in the model. These values are taken from epidemiological studies, which will have
used samples of patients to derive their estimates. Use of a sample introduces uncertainty into the estimate, which is summarized by the confidence interval or standard
error presented with the point estimate. Some pieces of data used in the model may
have very narrow confidence intervals indicating that the estimate is quite precise and
there is little uncertainty, while others may have wide confidence intervals indicating
high levels of uncertainty in the data. It is important to capture this parameter uncertainty in the model. Traditionally, the effect of parameter uncertainty on model conclusions has been tested by choosing high and low values for parameters (i.e., the best
and worst cases), substituting these values in the model and observing whether our
conclusions change. This method, called one-way sensitivity analysis and will not
characterize all parameter uncertainty as the conclusions depend on variability in
several parameters, not just one at a time. A multiway sensitivity analysis, with more
than one parameter varied at a time, is useful but the number of combinations esca-
lates with the number of parameters included. The best method for exploring parameter uncertainty is called probabilistic sensitivity analysis. This uses the information
from the confidence intervals provided with the original data to fit probability distributions to each model parameter. In this way, each parameter is described in terms of
a likely range of values it may take rather than discrete high, middle, and low numbers. Different types of parameter are likely to have different probable ranges for the
estimate. For example, estimates of length of stay will not fall below zero. An evaluation is run, say 1,000 times, using random or "Monte Carlo" resamples drawn for
each parameter from the range of likely values specified by the distribution. This
provides 1,000 estimates of the ICER, which when plotted on the cost-effectiveness
plane forms a cloud of points (i.e., ICERs). The advantage is that all parameter uncertainty has been carried forward to model results and can be used to give extra information to decision makers about how confident they can be in the conclusions of the

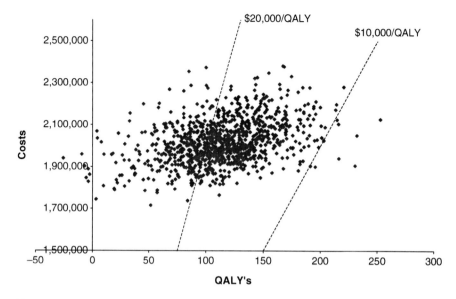

Fig. 19 The results of a probabilistic sensitivity analysis

model. This is the same principle as providing confidence intervals with an estimate of relative risk. These data in Fig. 19 show the results of a probabilistic sensitivity analysis of a single program compared with existing practice.

There are 1,000 separate estimates of the ICER represented by 1,000 points. The scatter arises from uncertainty in model parameters. These results are quite easy to interpret. There is a very small chance that this program will lead to health (i.e., QALY) losses as only seven points (count them) describe negative QALY outcomes, so the chance this program reduces QALYs is 7/1000 = 0.7%, the converse is that there is a 99.3% chance the QALY benefits are positive. There is no chance this program is cost saving, based on the input data used, as all points describe positive costs. To evaluate these data, we simply draw a straight line through the plane that describes a constant ceiling ratio. Here, we draw lines for $10,000 and $20,000 per QALY. The number of points that fall below these lines, divided by the total number of point (i.e., 1,000) represents the probability the intervention is cost-effective for each ceiling ratio. With a maximum willingness to pay for a QALYs of $10,000, we see only nine points below the ceiling ratio, so the probability the program is cost effective is 9/1000 = 0.9% and the probability that existing practice is cost effective is 100% minus 0.9% = 99.1%. The balance of probability suggests the best decision is to remain with existing practice. If we value health benefits at $20,000 then there are 820 points below the line, so now the probability the intervention is cost-effective is 82%, and the chances are that the best decision would be to adopt the new program. These are good examples of analysts using probabilistic sensitivity analysis to assess the cost-effectiveness of infection control programs [54–56].

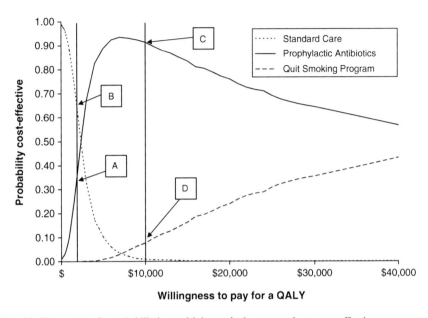

Fig. 20   The results of a probabilistic sensitivity analysis presented as a cost-effectiveness accept-ability curve

Without counting all the points, it is difficult to say what probability an inter-vention has of being cost-effective. If more than one intervention is being com-pared the plots can become confusing to interpret particularly if the clouds of points overlap. The results of a probabilistic sensitivity analysis are often rear-ranged and presented in the form of a cost-effectiveness acceptability curve (CEAC) rather than a scatter. Figure 20 shows a CEAC for an evaluation com-paring two alternative strategies to reduce the risk of surgical site infection to a baseline scenario where neither intervention is available. The first strategy is administration of prophylactic antibiotics, the second provision of a quit smok-ing program to patients 30 days prior to surgery. A CEAC is a graphical way of showing the probability that an intervention is cost-effective relative to its comparator(s). The horizontal axis measures the ceiling ratio (or the decision makers' willingness-to-pay for health benefits) and the vertical axis measures the probability, given the ceiling ratio, that the intervention is cost-effective. If decision makers are willing to pay only $2,000/QALY, then the probability that the administration of prophylactic antibiotics is cost-effective is 40% (Point A), the probability the quit smoking program is cost-effective is 0%, and the prob-ability that standard practice is cost-effective is 60% (Point B). However, if decision makers are willing to pay $10,000 per QALY then the probability that prophylactic antibiotics are cost-effective increases to 91% (Point C), the prob-ability that the quit smoking program is cost-effective rises to 8% (Point D), and the probability that standard practice is cost-effective falls to 1%. Note that the probabilities across the three options always sum to one. For decision makers, a summary of this analysis would be that if QALYs are valued at <$2,500 standard practice is the most likely to be the optimal choice, if QALYs are valued at >$2,500 then prophylactic antibiotics are most likely to be optimal and across the range of ceiling ratios considered here the quit smoking program is unlikely to be cost-effective.

Probabilistic sensitivity analysis is a powerful tool and can be used to find out whether we should do more studies in the future to reduce uncertainty in the decision at hand, if you want to read more about this topic have a look at Drummond [50] and Briggs [52].

4.2.5 Objective Five: Value Future Research

The presence of large amounts of uncertainty may result in decision makers choosing not to make a decision. Uncertainty can be reduced by collecting more data and so improving the decision. How much value there is in collecting more information on any given parameter depends on how influential the parameter is within the model and how much new information we would gain from the new data. Take the example, the use of silver-alloy catheters for the prevention of urinary tract infection in adult patients. Within this model, we might be very unsure about the mortality that is attributable to the infection and the effectiveness of these catheters in reducing risk of infection. Our estimate of attributable mortality comes from one observational study conducted in elderly patients. The design and conduct of a high quality prospective study that improves understanding of attributable mortality in a more general population would reduce uncertainty and make the decision easier. In contrast, if the estimate of how much catheters reduce risk of infection is derived from a metaanalysis of 25 good quality trials. Diverting research monies to another trial that will likely confirm the existing knowledge adds little additional information about the intervention, does little to reduce uncertainty, and is therefore of low value. Karl Claxton [57, 58] has written some good papers on this subject.

4.3 Important Features of an Economic Appraisal

A good quality economic appraisal will demonstrate a number of characteristics. Some of the major ones are described in this section.

Include all relevant options: It is important to make sure that all relevant options are included in the model; otherwise, we cannot make a good decision. If a program has already been shown to be most costly and less effective than something else then it can be excluded, but if we are not sure about this, then it should be considered in the model. The argument that we do not have good data about a program is not a good one. By excluding a relevant program, we are making a positive decision not to choose that program. The decision has not gone away just because we choose to ignore a program we know little about. The program should be included in a model with uncertainties appropriately described. The effect of these uncertainties can be carried forward and we can assess the value of collecting further data to reduce them. This framework is useful even when there is limited information available to inform a decision because it makes what it is that is not known about the decision explicit, rather than ignoring it just because there is no information.

Use the best available evidence: We must use the best evidence available to inform the decision model. If there are 12 studies that purport to measure the same parameter, such as the risk of mortality among patients with infection, then the merits of each study should be considered. Some of the studies may be poorly designed, and there may be threats to the validity of the conclusions. Others may be conducted in populations that are quite different from the one we are attempting to describe. There may only be a few studies that are useful and inform the decision at hand. Halton and Graves [59] made this point when they reviewed published models of the cost-effectiveness of interventions that reduce catheter-related BSI among ICU patients. They found that there was little critical appraisal of the quality of evidence used to inform model parameters. The answer is for analysts to use a systematic approach to select evidence. Nicola Cooper and her colleagues [60] reviewed the sources and the quality of the evidence used for decision models developed between 1997 and 2003 for a UK-based health technology assessment program. They modified and then applied a quality appraisal tool called the "Potential Hierarchies of Data Sources" developed by Doug Coyle [61]. Their conclusions were that decision models are informed by evidence from diverse sources and that this evidence should be quality assessed if policy agencies (i.e., the decision maker) are to make good decisions.

Consider final endpoints: It is important to consider final endpoints such as mortality or QALY outcomes. A cost-effectiveness model that only estimates the cost per infection avoided is useful, but not that useful. It can only tell us whether one program is productively efficient compared with others, at preventing infections. It will show the least cost method of preventing an infection. If we were comparing a program to reduce risk of urinary tract infection among maternity patients with the risk of bloodstream infection among the critically ill patients, it is clear that the benefits of preventing each type of infection are different. By translating the benefits of avoided infections into QALY gains, we can make a meaningful comparison. This also has the advantage of allowing comparisons with other parts of the health care sector such as cancer treatments and cardio vascular treatments, for example. Measuring outcomes in natural units, which are not QALYs (or life years gained), only informs productive efficiency and not allocative or economic efficiency.

Model the correct time period: The appropriate time period should be described by the model. If relevant costs and benefits are likely to accrue 3–6 months after discharge from hospital, then these must be captured. A model that stops when the patient leaves the hospital may omit outcomes that could change the conclusions. A new program to reduce risks of surgical site infection that does not describe patient outcomes after discharge may miss important events such as postdischarge infection, additional morbidity, and cost. Similarly, there is a long-term risk of mortality associated with bloodstream infection, and this should be described by the model. This is one of the key advantages of the modeling approach when compared with conducting cost-effectiveness alongside a clinical trial discussed at the start of this chapter.

Discount future costs and benefits: If costs and benefits occur in the future then these should be adjusted or discounted to a present value (i.e., today's value). The reason is that we prefer to have benefits now, rather than in the future, and would rather avoid paying costs now, when compared to in the future. Buying a house is a good example. We want all the benefits of the house now, and wish to delay paying the costs, and that is why we borrow money to finance our house. The alternative would be to live in a tent for 20 years while we save up the price of a house, when all the money is saved we buy it.

For health care decision making, we prefer health benefits now. If given a choice between discovering a cure for cancer today or in five years of time, the former would always be preferred. For this reason, we should deflate the value of health benefits that arise in the future to today's values. Similarly, we prefer to avoid paying for health care now, and so costs that arise in the future should be reduced in value, for a decision that is made today. There are examples of using discounting in the upcoming chapters, in particular Chap. 8.

4.4 Conclusions

In the context of infection control, modeling studies are likely to be more useful than adding an economic appraisal to a clinical trial of some new intervention. Modeling studies are certainly a multidisciplinary activity. Those who undertake them should choose an appropriate model structure, find the evidence required to inform the model and then evaluate the model appropriately. They should also be aware of heterogeneity and uncertainty and preferably use probabilistic sensitivity analyses as a means of exploring this uncertainty. They may also want to consider the value of collecting additional data in the future to improve the decision they are evaluating. Modeling is potentially powerful but studies should be of high quality and be carefully designed and executed.

Chapter 5
Changes Arising from the Adoption of Infection Control Programs

Preview

- The types of costs that arise from infection control programs are described and illustrated.
- The benefits that arise from infection control programs are described and illustrated.
- Some methods to measure the clinical effectiveness of infection control interventions are described.

5.1   Overview of the Major Changes

A new infection control program will lead to a different set of cost outcomes and will prevent infections among hospital patients. Some examples of summary cost outcomes, and how they were used to inform decision making were described in the previous chapter. Take for example the data in Table 7 in Chap. 4. We saw that for existing practice the costs were $8,777 but when Program 4 was adopted these increased to $10,520. These summary cost outcomes arise from two opposing forces. The resources used to implement and maintain a program must be measured and valued, and the cost savings that accrue from preventing cases of HAI should also be included. Also, and most important, is that infections are prevented, leading to an increase in health benefits. The example of Program 4 vs. Existing practice (Table 7 in Chap. 4) shows health benefits increasing from 19.47 to 19.52 QALYs. We use QALYs to measure health benefits because we take an extra welfarist view of economics (see Chap. 2). The health benefits arise from preventing infection among patients.

These changes all happen roughly at the same time, after the decision to implement infection control is taken. They are described next and then each of them is dealt with separately in their own chapter. Chapter 6 is about how to measure the costs of HAI, Chap. 7 is about how to measure the cost of implementing infection control, and Chap. 8 is about how to value the health benefits of preventing infections with QALYs.

N. Graves et al., *Economics and Preventing Healthcare Acquired Infection*,
DOI: 10.1007/978-0-387-72651-9_6, © Springer Science+Business Media, LLC 2009

The information in Fig. 21, which represents the cost-effectiveness plane described in Chaps. 3 and 4, shows one force pushing costs upward and the other pushing costs downwards. The increase in costs from developing, implementing, and maintaining the infection control program is $500,000. The cost savings that arise from avoided cases of HAI are valued at $800,000. The summary (or final) cost outcome (i.e., ΔC) from the "New Program" is a cost saving of $300,000, which is marked by the vertical double headed dashed arrow. Health benefits have also increased by ΔE because infections have been prevented, and these are marked with the horizontal double headed dashed arrow. Note that the cost savings accrue only because infections are prevented.

Under this scenario, the cost savings more than compensate the positive costs of the program and the decision maker is faced with the easy job of recommending the adoption of the program. This decision occupies Quadrant II of the cost-effectiveness

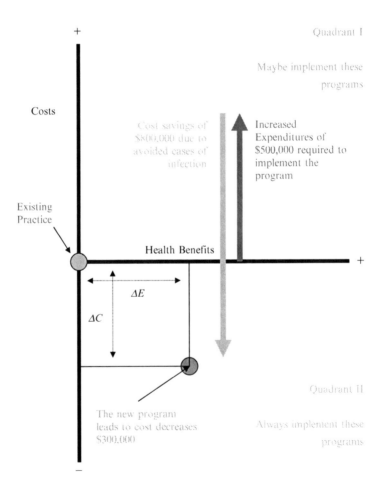

Fig. 21 How costs might change with more infection control (decrease overall)

plane (i.e., always implement the program) and is like Outcome 1 discussed in the Introduction to this book. Infection control is said to dominate existing practice because it leads to improved cost outcomes and improved health outcomes.

An alternate scenario is illustrated with Fig. 22 where the cost savings from infection-control do not compensate the cost increases. Implementing this program increases costs by $250,000 but leads to cost savings of only $100,000. The overall change in costs is positive $150,000 but health benefits are enjoyed as infections are prevented. A point in Quadrant I is reached and the adoption of this program might or might not be efficient (i.e., it could be the same as Outcome 2 or 3, described in the Introduction chapter). This depends on the ceiling ratio, or maximum willingness to pay for health benefits, used by decision makers and this was discussed in Chap. 3.

The methods used to measure the costs of HAI and so the potential cost savings from infection control are the subject of the next chapter, Chap. 6. The methods used to measure the costs of implementing infection control programs are the subject of Chap. 7. The methods used to value the health benefits that arise from preventing infections – the horizontal double headed dashed arrow – are the subject of Chap. 8. Before we embark on these three chapters, we have to think about how to measure the effectiveness of infection control programs, and this is the subject of the next section.

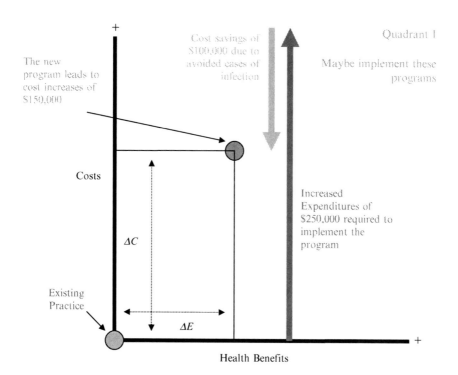

Fig. 22 How costs might change with more infection control (increase overall)

5.2   Changes to the Number of Infections

At the heart of infection control is whether or not the program is effective. An effective program will prevent infections and deliver health benefits (ΔE) and so move into the space to the right of the vertical axes drawn in Figs. 21 and 22. Some methods to measure whether an infection control program works, and if it does, how well it works, are described in the remainder of this chapter.

5.2.1   Epidemiological Studies

There is evidence to suggest that risks of infection will change with different clinical practices and interventions. Stefan Harbarth and colleagues [62] undertook a systematic review of 30 epidemiological studies of multimodal intervention studies and concluded that rates of healthcare acquired infections could be reduced by between 10% and 70% depending on setting, study design, baseline infection rates, and type of infection. Overall they suggest 20% of all healthcare acquired infections could be prevented by making changes to infection control practices. Implicit in this conclusion is that the there exists a true causal effect between an infection control intervention and the outcome. That is, we believe patients are protected from infections because of the application of infection-control and not for other reasons.

Epidemiological studies to measure this causal effect vary by how successfully bias, confounding, and other threats to validity are managed. The gold standard is a randomized controlled trial (RCT); however, these are expensive, time consuming, and often cause ethical problems. It is not acceptable to withhold an effective intervention from a patient who would benefit. Many infection control programs are not patient specific and benefit a group of patients, for instance a staff education program to improve compliance to hand hygiene and so randomizing individual patients is not possible. A solution is to randomize groups or clusters of patients but this design requires a complex study, which will take time to design, fund, and implement. This problem compounds when a rapid response, say, to an outbreak, is required. For these reasons, RCTs are often not practical. Instead, quasi-experimental designs that are either prospective or retrospective are used. They do not use randomization but still aim to find evidence for a true causal relationship between an intervention and the outcome.

Harris and colleagues [63] published a review of the use and interpretation of quasi-experimental designs for infectious diseases research. They highlight some of the problems of using quasi-experimental designs in infectious diseases and point out that some designs are better than others. Eight different types of study were organised in two categories: first are quasi-experimental study designs that do not use control groups, and second are quasi-experimental designs that use control groups and pretests. They identify a hierarchy among study designs with those in the second category found to be superior to those in the first. It may be the case that you need to design an epidemiological study, experimental or other, to find out whether expanding infection control is effective or not and for this we recommend you assemble the right mix of researchers and clinically trained individuals.

5.2.2 Synthesizing Existing Evidence

An alternative to setting up your own prospective study is to use existing research findings that describe the effectiveness of a given infection control strategy. A traditional literature review uses informal or subjective methods to select and then interpret evidence. The results are normally presented as a narrative and findings are summarized in tables. These types of review are commonly found at the start of PhD theses, grant applications, and journal articles. They demonstrate that the author has a good grasp of the literature and understands the topic in hand. They provide an individual interpretation a particular health issue or program. A systematic review is quite different. The authors follow a predefined protocol and their objective is to provide the definitive synthesis of the current data. A review must be reproducible by others who would follow research methods that have been written down in a protocol. The Cochrane Collaboration (http://www.cochrane.org/) manages a large number of systematic reviews on a wide range of health topics. Two relevant Cochrane reviews are described in Panel 4.

The Cochrane Collaboration published a handbook that provides guidance for those wishing to conduct their own systematic review [66]. There are seven steps for completing a review:

Step 1. Formulate the problem: The question needs to be relevant and interesting and authors should clarify which patient populations they wish to gather information about, the interventions to be compared, and the outcome measures to be reported.

Step 2. Locate and select epidemiological studies: The primary source of evidence will be electronic databases, such as the United States National Library of Medicine. Standardized medical subject headings should be used (see www.nlm.nih.gov/mesh/) to search with and the combinations of search terms reported so that other can reproduce the search. It is important for the search to be specific enough (i.e., it should return a manageable number of studies, a search that finds 5,000 articles is not useful) and sensitive enough (i.e., it must locate all known important papers). In addition to interrogating electronic databases, other search strategies can be used such as internet searching, consultation with key researchers and professional associations for unpublished data, and manual searches of conference proceedings and journals indexes. Studies should be selected based on predefined inclusion and exclusion criteria such as time frame (e.g., 1995–2007) age groups (e.g., adults only), key diagnoses and interventions (e.g., catheter-related blood stream infection). Often a review of the abstract is sufficient to determine whether a study should be included. A good practice is that two reviewers assess every study independently and then compare notes afterwards and decide which are eligible. Notes should also be kept on why studies are included or excluded.

A systematic review - isolation measures for infants with candida

Mohan, Eddama and Weisman [64] undertook a systematic review of patient isolation measures for infants with Candida colonization or infection. The objective was to determine the effect of patient isolation measures for infants with Candida colonization or infection as an adjunct to routine infection control measures on the transmission of Candida to other infants in the neonatal unit. The authors concluded:

> ➤ there is no evidence to either support or refute the use of patient isolation measures (single room isolation or cohorting) in neonates with Candida colonization or infection.
> ➤ despite the evidence for transmission of Candida by direct or indirect contact and evidence of cross-infection by health care workers, no standard policy of patient isolation measures beyond routine infection control measures exists in the neonatal unit.
> ➤ there is an urgent need to research the role of patient isolation measures for preventing transmission of Candida in the neonatal unit.

A systematic review – prophylaxis for ceserean delivery

Smaill & Hofmeyr [65] undertook a systematic review of antibiotic prophylaxis for ceserean section. The objective was to assess the effects of prophylactic antibiotic treatment on infectious complications in women undergoing cesarean delivery. The authors included 81 trials in their review and found:

> ➤ the use of prophylactic antibiotics in women undergoing cesarean section substantially reduced the incidence of episodes of fever, endometritis, wound infection, urinary tract infection and serious infection after cesarean section.
> ➤ the reduction in the risk of endometritis with antibiotics was substantial and similar for elective, non-elective and then all patients.
> ➤ wound infections were also reduced: for elective cesarean section, for non-elective cesarean section and for all patients.
> ➤ the reduction of endometritis by two thirds to three quarters and a decrease in wound infections justifies a policy of recommending prophylactic antibiotics to women undergoing elective or non-elective cesarean section.

Panel 4 Two examples of published systemic reviews

Step 3. Assess the quality of each study: Once the list of eligible studies is decided they can be assessed for quality. At this stage, it is sometimes useful to blind the studies by removing all citation details. Reviewers sometimes use checklists to help decide whether epidemiological studies have minor or serious flaws. Some examples are the "Effective Public Health Practice Project – Quality Assessment

Tool for Quantitative Studies" available from Faculty of Applied Health Sciences, University of Waterloo, (http://www.ahs.uwaterloo.ca/~manske/Presentations/ UNB%20workshop/QADictionary2003.pdf), and the Scottish Intercollegiate Guidelines Network tool (http://www.sign.ac.uk/methodology/checklists.html). It is important to have epidemiological expertise available for this step, as some studies may be excluded from the review based on the quality of the epidemiological methods reported. In some cases, it is necessary to clarify facts with the authors of the studies with an e-mail or phone call.

Step 4. Collecting data: The information you need to collect from the studies should be predefined and data collection forms checked with pilot studies. Two independent reviewers should collect data from each study and then compare the results. Differences should be resolved by returning to the articles or contacting the original authors of the study.

Step 5. Analyze and presenting results: A systematic review will sometimes find different studies that have been designed to measure the same outcome. The results from a collection of studies can be combined to provide a quantitative summary of all the data using a process called meta-analysis. This is appropriate when there are no obvious differences between the studies and outcomes are measured in similar ways. A meta-analysis will show the combined estimate of effect for a number of studies, it will show how precise the effect is and so capture uncertainty around the mean effect, and it allows an opportunity to describe heterogeneity and bias. Effect size and precision are displayed with a Forest plot. An example is presented from Ramritu [67] and colleagues in Fig. 23.

The objective was to compare the effectiveness of chlorhexidine/silver sulfadiazine-impregnated central venous catheters vs. nonimpregnated catheters for preventing catheter-related blood stream infection. Each study is represented by a black square, the bigger the square the more weight that study has on the summary estimate, and a horizontal line that marks the 95% confidence intervals. Note the bigger squares have shorter horizontal lines. The pooled or summary estimate is shown as a diamond. These data in Fig. 23 show the risk of catheter-related blood stream infection is reduced by 44% if chlorhexidine/silver sulfadiazine-impregnated central venous catheters are used compared with nonimpregnated catheters. Because the 95% confidence interval does not cross 1, the result is statistically significant.

Step 6. Interpret results: Authors should be very clear about what they have found. They should consider uncertainty in their findings that might arise from say excluding some studies (e.g., those published before 2000 or those conducted in small hospitals), publication bias, or concerns about the quality of some studies. Whether the findings are useful is also important. The review might have filled a major gap in the evidence base or the evidence synthesized might have just confirmed existing beliefs. There might also be other useful data that were not primary outcomes but were still collected, such as costs, the frequency of adverse events, and what baseline practice is for each study.

Step 7. Improve and update reviews: A review is an ongoing responsibility and the authors are required to update the review to capture new evidence as it become available.

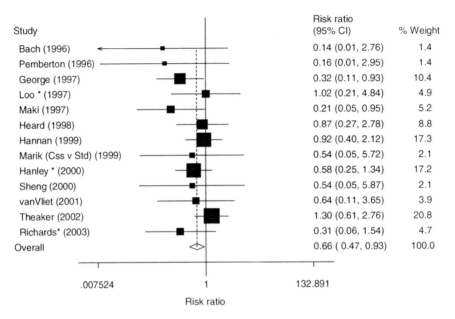

Fig. 23 Forest plot of the effectiveness chlorhexidine/silver sulfadiazine-impregnated central venous catheters vs. nonimpregnated catheters for preventing catheter related blood stream infection

Each step of the systematic review process is carefully described and documented so that others can reproduce the results in different settings or in future time periods. The results of a systematic review should be less biased and valid compared with other approaches to summarizing scientific evidence. Cynthia Multrow [68], who edited the Cochrane handbook, suggests:

> Systematic literature reviews including meta-analyses are invaluable scientific activities. The rationale for such reviews is well established. Health care providers, researchers, and policy makers are inundated with unmanageable amounts of information; they need systematic reviews to efficiently integrate existing information and provide data for rational decision making.

An advantage of systematic reviews and meta-analysis are that existing data can be exploited, and prospective data collection via potentially expensive _epidemiological studies avoided. A careful and systematic approach can reduce bias when compared with nonsystematic approaches. They can provide reliable information for decision making by demonstrating whether some intervention is effective. They are not a trivial undertaking exercise and anyone considering undertaking a systematic review should assemble a team with specialist skills in epidemiology and biostatistics and consider clearing their diary for 6–8 months. They should also consult an academic librarian. Even after completion, the results may still be inconclusive, the evidence found may have been poor quality, and so was screened out of the review and decision-makers will only be made aware of what they do not know. Matthias Egger and his colleagues published a series of papers in the Education section of the BMJ that covers many important aspects of systematic reviews and meta-analyses [69–74].

Making estimates of the number of infections prevented by infection control is incredibly useful but not sufficient to complete the economic argument for prevention. Both the cost implications of preventing infections and the value of the health benefits from preventing infections need to be quantified. These tasks are the subject of the next three chapters.

5.3 Conclusions

Infection control will change cost outcomes. Some costs, such as those incurred designing, implementing, and monitoring infection control programs will increase. Others such as the costs of treating the cases of infection will be saved and so will lead to cost reductions. To some extent these two opposing forces cancel each other out. Infection control can lead to an overall increase or decrease in cost outcomes. Infection control will also prevent cases of HAI. Prospective epidemiological studies can be designed to measure how effective a given program might be, but these are major undertakings and must be designed carefully to avoid biased results. An alternative way to investigate whether infection control is effective is to synthesize the published literature using a systematic review method and the pooling of results in meta-analysis. This is a potentially powerful tool but can be time consuming and complex.

Chapter 6
Measuring the Cost of Healthcare Acquired Infections

Preview

- We discuss why estimates of the costs of HAI are made.
- The differences between the accountancy and economics approaches to costing are illustrated.
- The relevance of the different approaches for economic appraisal is discussed.
- The different epidemiological methods available to investigate associations between HAI and cost outcomes are reviewed.

6.1   Why Data on the Cost of HAI are Useful

Data on the costs generated by HAI are useful for two purposes. The first is to highlight the size of the problem. An estimate of how much these infections cost a healthcare system can make politicians and decision-makers sit up and take notice. The second use for cost data is to update our understanding of how costs will change with the adoption of extra infection control, thereby providing some positive economic insight for allocating resources to preventing infection.

As discussed in Chap. 5, the costs of HAI are an important part of the overall change to costs (ΔC) that will arise with the adoption of additional infection control interventions. Consideration of ΔC alongside the change in health benefits (ΔE) forms the basis for economic appraisal. This framework can be used to allocate resources within an infection control budget to get the best value for money. It can also be used to support arguments for additional infection control. Costs must be estimated appropriately to make valid economic arguments. This highlights the importance of collecting good cost data.

N. Graves et al., *Economics and Preventing Healthcare Acquired Infection*,
DOI: 10.1007/978-0-387-72651-9_7, © Springer Science+Business Media, LLC 2009

6.2   Defining and Measuring Costs of HAI

Cost data can be presented and interpreted in a number of ways. If costs are not
handled properly when considering the (economic) question of allocating resources
to infection control, then erroneous conclusions will result. To understand the cost
of HAI, a distinction must be made between the two quite separate disciplines of
cost accountancy and economics. The current literature on the costs of HAI tends
to view cost through the eyes of a cost accountant, and these estimates are not useful for economic appraisal. The best estimates can only emerge using an economist's interpretation.

Before embarking on a comparison of the two approaches to measuring costs the
differences between a fixed and variable cost are defined in Panel 5. It is important
to understand these differences.

6.2.1   The Cost Accountant's Method

An accountant who works for a hospital is responsible for planning, monitoring,
and reporting expenditures in a given period, normally a 12-month budgeting cycle.
They aim to keep the organization financially solvent and recover all expenditures
by charging the payers for healthcare for the treatments and services supplied. This
is the same regardless of whether the payer is the government, an insurance company, or the patient. This process is relatively straightforward for fluids, pharma-
ceuticals, drains, and other consumable items used by patients. These items can be
counted, the purchase price is easy to obtain, and their use can be recorded. Variable
costs might be counted up, item by item, and added to a patient's bill. Expenditures
on salaries or hospital overheads (i.e., fixed costs) cannot be billed to patients in
this way. This is because fixed costs are often used jointly in production. There is
not one doctor for one patient or one heating system for one patient. Fixed costs are
often used by many patients over the course of one 12-month budget cycle. The
accountant records expenditure on these items and finds some measure of usage
that can be subsequently attributed to patients for the purpose of cost recovery.
Some units of usage are bed days, physician consultations, and number of radio-
logical investigations. They then calculate a cost per unit, which is used for patient
billing purposes.

For example, the total overhead costs of running the hospital such as maintenance, heating, lighting, insurance, cleaning, and IT systems might be calculated
and then allocated evenly across the total number of bed days supplied in a year to
give a cost per bed day. The longer patients stay in hospital the more of the overhead they pay. The expenditures associated with an MRI scanner will be allocated
on a cost per scan basis across all the patients who have an MRI scan. This makes
sense as the people who enjoy the benefits of the expenditure pay for it. Bills are
produced for each patient according to the treatments and services that have been

Time Frame

The period of time relevant to the decision about adopting infection control must be known. Infection control is normally funded from a 12 month budget. A decision maker will be interested in the additional infection control they can implement given this budget. We seek to understand which costs can and cannot change within the decision makers 12 month time frame.

Fixed costs	Variable costs
Expenditures that cannot be escaped within the 12 month time frame are fixed costs to the decision maker.	Expenditures that can be escaped within the 12 month time frame are variable costs to the decision maker.
Examples:	Examples:

Fixed costs

Examples:

o A doctor is employed on a two year contract. Infection rates fall and so they are less busy. The costs of employing the doctor cannot be changed as they are protected by their employment contract.

o A new IT system is installed in the hospital and will be used for 7 years before it is replaced. Infection rates fall but the costs of IT cannot be changed.

o A new ward was built to deal with patients that have long lengths of stay. Infection rates fall and there are fewer patients with long stays and so the new ward is not busy. The costs of the building cannot be escaped. The costs of heating, lighting, cleaning and maintenance still have to be met.

Variable costs

Examples:

o Dressings and syringes are ordered by the clinical nurse manager every week based on how busy the hospital has been. Infection rates fall, the size of the order is reduced and so costs are saved.

o Agency nurses and doctors are paid an hourly rate based on occupancy and how sick the patients are. Infection rates fall, the number of agency staff hours is reduced and costs are saved.

o An MRSA outbreak means that patients have to be isolated in single rooms. Some of these patients are moved into a neighbouring hospital with spare single rooms. The receiving hospital is paid $3000 for every bed day used. MRSA outbreaks are reduced and these costs are saved.

Panel 5 The difference between fixed and variable cost

provided. By following these methods, accountants will recover all expenditures, and the organization remains financially viable. These data in Table 8 illustrate an example of the cost-accountants method of allocating expenditure. The total annual expenditure for this hospital is $5M. The hospital manager makes expenditures of $500,000 per annum for the doctor's salaries, and these are allocated across the total number of consultations supplied in this time frame (i.e., 1,000, see Table 8). Therefore, the expenditure to be recovered from each consultation with a doctor is $500 (i.e., $500,000 divided by 1,000). The expenditures for nursing staff are $1.5M, and these are to be recovered based on 15,000 units of nursing workload, which are recorded on the wards throughout the year. The $1.5M expenditures made for overheads are spread across the 2,000 bed days supplied and so on. This process makes patients (or those who pay for them) accountable for the costs of their care. The mechanism of allocating these costs to the 30 patients treated at the hospital in this 12-month period, based on this method, is illustrated in Table 9.

Patient 1 required 18 consultations with a doctor. The expenditure that has to be recovered to ensure the hospital remains financially viable per consultation is $500 (see Table 8). This gives an allocated cost of $9,000 for this cost item for Patient 1. They also use 300 workload units of nurse time and the allocated cost per unit is $100, giving a cost of $3,000 for this cost item. This process of allocating costs by some surrogate measure of usage continues (i.e., 40 bed days, 35 radiology tests, and 20 path tests) until we get to consumables, which are not allocated but simply counted for each patient. The market price of consumables is then attached. The total of the costs are calculated in the final column of Table 9. The total costs for patient 1 is $106,499.

Using these data, we can calculate average costs per patient. It may be tempting to use these figures to estimate the cost of HAI. Look back at Table 9, Patients 1–20 did not get an infection during their stay. The total cost of treating these patients was $2,375,009 giving an average cost per patient of $118,750 (i.e., $2,375,009 divided by 20). Patients 21–30 did acquire an infection. The total cost of treating

Table 8 Expenditures for a 12 month budgetary cycle and measures for allocating expenditures

	Expenditures made by hospital	Allocation unit	Total of allocation unit	Cost per allocation unit
Doctors[a]	$500,000	Consultations	1,000	$500
Nurses[a]	$1,500,000	Units of nursing workload	15,000	$100
General over-heads[a]	$1,500,000	Bed days	2,000	$750
Radiology[a]	$250,000	# investigations	1,000	$250
Pathology[a]	$750,000	# tests	2,000	$375
Consumables[b]	$500,000	N/A	N/A	N/A
Total	$5,000,000			

[a]Fixed costs
[b]Variable costs are based on what the individual patient uses

Table 9 The result of a costing exercise for 30 patients based on cost-accounting methods

Number of the allocation units used by each patient (allocated costs in brackets)

	Doctors	Nurses	Overheads	Radiology	Pathology	Consumables	Total
Pat. 1	18 ($9,000)	300 ($30,000)	40 ($30,000)	35 ($8750)	20 ($7,500)	$21,249	$106,499
Pat. 2	11 ($5,500)	150 ($15,000)	20 ($15,000)	17 ($4250)	86 ($32,250)	$5,085	$77,085
Pat. 3	10 ($5,000)	150 ($15,000)	20 ($15,000)	40 ($10000)	72 ($27,000)	$12,527	$84,527
Pat. 4	27 ($13,500)	405 ($40,500)	54 ($40,500)	16 ($4000)	84 ($31,500)	$5,061	$135,061
Pat. 5	10 ($5,000)	150 ($15,000)	20 ($15,000)	17 ($4250)	88 ($33,000)	$3,564	$75,814
Pat. 6	15 ($7,500)	120 ($12,000)	16 ($12,000)	35 ($8750)	85 ($31,875)	$8,716	$80,841
Pat. 7	41 ($20,500)	615 ($61,500)	82 ($61,500)	17 ($4250)	22 ($8,250)	$9,289	$165,289
Pat. 8	10 ($5,000)	150 ($15,000)	20 ($15,000)	35 ($8750)	24 ($9,000)	$778	$53,528
Pat. 9	15 ($7,500)	225 ($22,500)	30 ($22,500)	42 ($10500)	20 ($7,500)	$2,750	$73,250
Pat. 10	12 ($6,000)	180 ($18,000)	24 ($18,000)	33 ($8250)	42 ($15,750)	$22,736	$88,736
Pat. 11	26 ($13,000)	480 ($48,000)	64 ($48,000)	43 ($10750)	40 ($15,000)	$13,231	$147,981
Pat. 12	13 ($6,500)	345 ($34,500)	46 ($34,500)	25 ($6250)	95 ($35,625)	$20,821	$138,196
Pat. 13	19 ($9,500)	375 ($37,500)	50 ($37,500)	27 ($6750)	66 ($24,750)	$11,694	$127,694
Pat. 14	22 ($11,000)	330 ($33,000)	44 ($33,000)	18 ($4500)	79 ($29,625)	$8,864	$119,989
Pat. 15	23 ($11,500)	345 ($34,500)	46 ($34,500)	40 ($10000)	94 ($35,250)	$13,799	$139,549
Pat. 16	23 ($11,500)	345 ($34,500)	46 ($34,500)	37 ($9250)	66 ($24,750)	$22,207	$136,707
Pat. 17	30 ($15,000)	450 ($45,000)	60 ($45,000)	40 ($10000)	68 ($25,500)	$11,731	$152,231
Pat. 18	23 ($11,500)	345 ($34,500)	46 ($34,500)	35 ($8750)	99 ($37,125)	$14,774	$141,149
Pat. 19	14 ($7,000)	390 ($39,000)	52 ($39,000)	23 ($5750)	75 ($28,125)	$881	$119,756
Pat. 20	32 ($16,000)	842 ($84,200)	64 ($48,000)	22 ($5500)	51 ($19,125)	$38,302	$211,127
Pat. 21	32 ($16,000)	754 ($75,400)	64 ($48,000)	36 ($9000)	24 ($9,000)	$25,020	$182,420
Pat. 22	24 ($12,000)	705 ($70,500)	20 ($15,000)	24 ($6000)	75 ($28,125)	$32,854	$164,479
Pat. 23	23 ($11,500)	685 ($68,500)	18 ($13,500)	21 ($5250)	82 ($30,750)	$22,558	$152,058

(continued)

Table 9 (continued)

Number of the allocation units used by each patient (allocated costs in brackets)

	Doctors	Nurses	Overheads	Radiology	Pathology	Consumables	Total
Pat. 24	12 ($6,000)	875 ($87,500)	24 ($18,000)	40 ($10000)	54 ($20,250)	$30,107	$171,857
Pat. 25	18 ($9,000)	754 ($75,400)	36 ($27,000)	31 ($7750)	97 ($36,375)	$17,601	$173,126
Pat. 26	80 ($40,000)	854 ($85,400)	160 ($120,000)	60 ($15000)	55 ($20,625)	$37,602	$318,627
Pat. 27	90 ($45,000)	987 ($98,700)	180 ($135,000)	41 ($10250)	67 ($25,125)	$27,154	$341,229
Pat. 28	105 ($52,500)	951 ($95,100)	210 ($157,500)	44 ($11000)	75 ($28,125)	$34,594	$378,819
Pat. 29	126 ($63,000)	869 ($86,900)	252 ($189,000)	56 ($14000)	100 ($37,500)	$7,539	$397,939
Pat. 30	96 ($48,000)	874 ($87,400)	192 ($144,000)	50 ($12500)	95 ($35,625)	$16,913	$344,438
Total	1000 ($500,000)	15000 ($1,500,000)	2000 ($1,500,000)	1000 ($250000)	2000 ($750,000)	$500,000	$5,000,000

these patients was $2,624,991 giving an average cost per patient of $262,499 (i.e., $2,624,991 divided by 10). They used more resources during their stay and their costs are greater.

A naïve and misleading interpretation of these data is to compare the average cost per infected patient ($118,750) and the average cost per uninfected patient ($262,499) and attribute the difference ($262,499 less $118,750 = $143,749) to the infection. This, multiplied by the ten cases of infection observed at the hospital, gives an estimate of the cost of HAI to this hospital of $1,437,486. These data are not suitable for economic appraisal or informing decision making for infection control. Accounting data cannot be used in this way to make economic arguments. The purpose of cost accounting data is to keep the hospital financially viable.

The implication is that $1,437,486 could be saved annually by eradicating HAI. To understand why this number is misleading, we must think like an economist. Accountants and hospital administrators use allocation methods, quite appropriately, to recover expenditure. However, the main reason the cost of infection is measured is to argue for additional infection control programs. This represents a reallocation of scarce resources toward infection control, which is an economics question (see Chap. 1).

The accountancy approach ignores the costs of increased investment which will be required for additional infection control (the cost of implementing infection control programs is discussed in Chap. 7, and is an important consideration in this decision). The accountancy approach also fails to consider what costs actually change with fewer infections. Whether costs actually change with rates of infection depend on whether they are fixed or variable in the time frame within which decisions are made. As previously stated, it is very important to understand the difference between fixed and variable costs. The economists approach to looking at the cost of infection takes into account both these points when exploring how costs will change with a decision to increase infection control.

6.2.2   The Economist's Method

An economist does a cost analysis and finds that, during the next 12 months, few costs can be saved if rates of infection are reduced. The reason is that none of the employment contracts with the staff can be broken and the administrators are unwilling to shut down any part of the hospital. The only costs that will change with more infection control are savings from the consumable items (i.e., variable costs) that would have been required to treat the consequences of infection. They find that doctors and nurses will be less busy, fewer radiology and pathology investigations will be required, and beds will be empty because the length of stay has reduced for some patients. The main comment is that few cash expenditures are saved. Within the 12 months time frame relevant to the decision about increasing infection control, all costs are fixed, except consumables that are variable. The economist suggests that the capacity made available by infection control – the time of the doctors and nurses and the capacity to do pathology and radiology tests and the bed days – are valuable and should be redeployed for another use. This argument is made using a series of diagrams illustrated in Figs. 24–26.

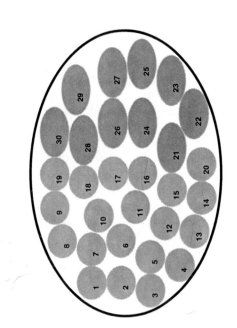

Existing Practice

The oval represents the hospital with total annual costs of $5M. Ninety percent of these expenditures are fixed costs that must be paid regardless of the number of patients treated – you can work this out from the data in Table 8.

Thirty patients (numbered 1-30) are treated in a year at a total cost of $5M.

Patients 21 to 30 get an infection and have a longer stay than patients 1-20 who remain free of infection.

Patients 21 to 30 take up a greater proportion each of the capacity of the hospital (almost half) as they have a longer stay in hospital.

Fig. 24 Hospital costs and throughput prior to infection control

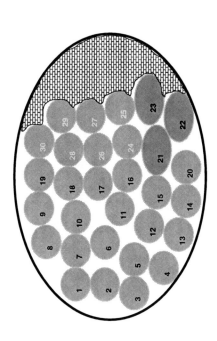

<u>A decision is made to increase Infection Control</u>

An additional infection control program is introduced, increasing total costs by $500,000 to $5.5M.

Under the improved infection control arrangements only three patients get an infection (# 21 #22 and #23). Patients 24 to 30 are now protected from HAI.

The only expenditures saved are some consumables for patients 24 to 30 as they do not have infection. The costs of consumables for these patients fall from $171,510 to $71,510, a saving of $100,000.

Thirty patients are still treated in a year for a new total cost of $5.4M ($5.5M less the saving of $100,000).

Patients 24 to 30 now have shorter stays in hospital. There is spare capacity in the hospital in the form of available bed days, the doctors and nurses are less busy and fewer diagnostic services required.

Fig. 25 Hospital costs and throughput after implementation of infection control

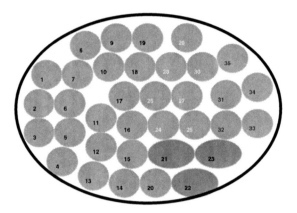

Costs have changed

The spare capacity is re-deployed and five new patients are treated (#31 to #35). The
increase to variable costs for each new patient is $10,000 per case. Costs increase by $50,000

Total costs increase from $5.4M to $5.45M.

The payers for health care now re-imburse the hospital $150,000 for each new patient
treated (patients #31 to #35).

Revenue rises by $750,000 and is used to offset total costs, which fall from $5.45M to $4.7M.

The net change in cost from additional infection control (ΔC) is $5M less $4.7M = negative
$300,000.

Look back at Figure 21 (Chapter 5) to see these data plotted on the cost-effectiveness plane.

Fig. 26   Hospital costs and throughput after implementation of infection control and new admissions

Figure 24 shows that prior to the implementation of an infection control program, 30 patients (numbered 1–30) are treated for an annual expenditure of $5
million. The oval boundary shows the capacity of the hospital; it is currently running at full capacity as there is no space to admit any new patients. Patients 21–30
get an infection and have longer stays than the other patients, who remain free of
infection. That is why the infected patients take up almost half of the capacity of
the hospital. Ninety percent of the $5M of expenditure are fixed costs that must be
paid regardless of the number of patients treated, and this can be worked out from
the data in Table 8.

Figure 25 shows what happens after a decision is made to implement an infection
control program. Risks are reduced and only three patients get an infection (number
21–23). Patients 24–30 have been protected from an infection they would have
acquired without the extra infection control program. The cost of implementing the
infection control program is $500,000, and so the total costs of running the hospital
rise to $5.5M. The only expenditures saved are the consumables not used to treat

the infections among patients 24–30 and so costs fall from $171,510 to $71,510, a cash saving of $100,000. This results in 30 patients being treated for $5.4M ($5.5M less the cash saving of $100,000). Patients 24–30 now have a shorter stay in hospital and there is some spare capacity in the form of empty beds and staffs are less busy than before. The spare capacity is marked by the brick pattern in Fig. 25.

The hospital administrators redeploy the spare capacity toward treating five additional patients illustrated by Fig. 26. Patients 31–35 are new admissions, which are only possible because of the infection control program. This causes variable costs to raise by $10,000 per patient but the payers of healthcare fund an additional $150,000 per patient for their treatments. Overall expenditures have increased from $5.4M to $5.45 million because of the new admissions but they attract additional revenues of $750,000, which offset total costs to a figure of $4.7M. The final change to cost outcomes (ΔC) is $5M less $4.7M = negative $300,000. Or in other words the hospital saves $300,000. These data are plotted in Fig. 21 (Chap. 5).

6.2.3   Differences Between the Cost Accounting and Economics Methods

The interpretation of the accountancy data in Table 9 suggest the cost of infection was $1,437,486. The conclusion is misleading because it is based on an assumption that all costs are variable (i.e., that fixed expenditures can be avoided when infections are prevented). The cost and effectiveness of any proposed infection control strategy is also ignored. The economist estimated that cost savings of $300,000 would actually be achieved by the hospital. This estimate takes into account that many costs are fixed within the time period for decision making, the program is itself costly, and not every case of infection can be prevented. Even though many costs are fixed, resources can be redeployed to other valuable activities such as making new admissions. Evidence from the literature supports the economist's approach. Roberts et al. [75] found that 84% and Plowman et al. [76] found that 89% of the costs of hospital care are fixed in the short term.

An important part of describing how costs change with more infection control is therefore the number of bed days released. The example illustrated by the economist's method (Sect. 6.2.2) shows why this is the case. Because most of the costs of running a hospital are fixed, it is the value of the capacity released by infection control that is important. A journal article by Graves provides an opportunity to consider these ideas again [4]. We would strongly recommend against using accounting data to estimate the costs of infection. They are not designed for the purpose of making economic arguments and will lead to poor decision making.

A good study of the economic costs of infection, therefore, requires that multiple pieces of data are collected. The points below are a summary of the data a cost analyst requires:

- They must understand the time frame within which decisions are to be made about infection control. Most budgets in a hospital cover a period of 12 months. After that time the budget may be renegotiated.
- They must understand the contractual obligations to expenditures made by the hospital for this period. The costs that are fixed and variable in the time frame for decision making must be known.
- They need data on how effective the program is at reducing rates of infection, so they can predict the number of infections that will be avoided if the decision is made.
- They must estimate the costs of implementing the program because infection control is a costly activity.
- The variable costs associated with treating the consequences of infection and the extra length of stay associated with treating the consequences of infection must also be known.

6.3   Estimating the Increase in Length of Stay due to HAI

The arguments made in this chapter show how important it is to identify the extra length of stay – and other cost outcomes such as variable costs – that arise from infection. This has been the subject of many hundreds of research papers since the 1950s. Studies have been conducted in over 30 countries [77] and a range of epidemiological methods have been used. The methods used to attribute length of stay and other cost outcomes to HAI are considered next.

There are many reasons why patients stay in hospital longer than might be expected given their primary diagnosis. The incidence of infection is a likely candidate but other intrinsic and external factors certainly contribute. To understand the cost of infection, the analyst must know the independent effect of HAI on length of stay, and this implies the effects of other factors have been taken into account. To illustrate this point, we show some information collected from patients admitted to two hospitals in Australia [78]. Data were collected on length of stay outcomes and factors that impact on length of stay, for 4,357 hospitalized patients. These data are summarized into four groups: the 4,230 patients who did not acquire an infection; the 27 patients who acquired a lower respiratory tract infection (LRTI); the 59 patients with a healthcare acquired urinary tract infection (UTI); and 41 patients with an "other" site of infection of which the majority where skin infections. Mean values for selected variables in this set of data are presented in Table 10.

Length of stay in hospital is much lower for patients who did not have an infection (mean = 4.8 days) compared with those who did (mean = 15.19 for LRTI, 14.86 for UTI and 15.49 for other). Variable costs (i.e., the costs of consumable items) were also much lower for those without infection. There is evidence in Table 10 that patients may have stayed longer and incurred greater variable cost regardless of whether they had an infection or not. For example, patients with infection were on average older, fewer were discharged to their home, or classified as "self caring

Table 10 Mean values for selected variable collected from 4,425 patients

Variables	No HAI (n = 4,260)	LRTI (n = 27)	UTI (n = 59)	Other (n = 41)
Cost and mortality outcomes				
Length of hospital stay (days)	4.8	15.19	14.86	15.49
Variable costs – total ($)	121.77	1097	176.93	1142.61
Died in hospital	2%	22%	14%	17%
Patient characteristics				
Age on admission (years)	57	67	72	65
Self caring prior to admission	71%	54%	39%	59%
Discharged Home	95%	70%	75%	71%
Adverse events during admission				
Fall	1%	7%	10%	5%
Cardiac arrest	2%	22%	14%	17%
Pressure ulcer	3%	26%	14%	15%
Faecally incontinent	5%	30%	29%	22%
Anaemic	38%	93%	71%	71%
Comorbidities				
Chronic obstructive pulmonary disease	11%	26%	20%	12%
Congestive heart failure	6%	15%	14%	10%
Diabetes	16%	33%	34%	17%
Ever had a stroke	7%	11%	20%	20%
Hypertension	35%	44%	51%	41%

prior to admission." These facts might indicate they were less healthy prior to the admission and so more likely to have an extended stay. Those with infection suffered more adverse events during the admission such as falls and pressure ulcers. These events, regardless of infection, might explain longer stays in hospital. Comorbidities such as heart failure and diabetes were more frequent among those with infection and may extend length of stay independent of the effect of infection. These data show there are many reasons why those with an infection might have stayed in hospital longer than those without, regardless of the infection. The relationship between infection and length of stay is likely to be confounded by other factors.

Examples of crude comparisons between those with HAI and those without can be found in the literature. An inexperienced analyst might deduct the mean length of stay for patients with LRTI (15.19 days) from the mean length of stay for those without HAI (4.8 days) and conclude the extra stay due to infection is 10.39 days. These estimates have no value for decision making because other factors likely to affect length of stay have not been controlled. The bias is positive and 10.39 is an overestimate of the effect of HAI on length of stay. Research methods are available to estimate the independent effects of infection on cost outcomes. These fall in one of two categories depending on whether attempts are made to control for confounding within the "design of the study" or whether "statistical modeling techniques" are employed.

6.3.1 Design Approaches

*Concurrent attribution studies:*These studies rely on experts to review data on the patient's admission with the goal of identifying by how much HAI prolonged stay in hospital and increased the use of other health care resources. These judgments are typically made by physicians or nurse infection control experts and sometimes hospital epidemiologists are involved. Critics of this method argue the results are unreliable and that different observers or the same observer, in different time periods, will not make consistent estimates [79]. Some believe these studies are likely to underestimate the costs of HAI as the surveyor judges extra cost conservatively [80, 81]. To make the method rigorous, Wakefield et al. [82] proposed the "standardized case review protocol." This required trained staff to follow carefully prepared protocols. They assessed each day of the patient's hospital stay according to whether it was:

- Attributable to the reason for admission
- Jointly attributable to the reason for admission and the HAI
- Attributable to the HAI alone

The approach was tested by Gertman and Restuccia [83] and Rishpon et al., [84] who found high levels of interviewer agreement. The conclusion was that estimates depend on the quality of the data included in the patient's records.

Comparative attribution studies: These vary by the sophistication of their design. Unmatched (crude) comparisons have been discussed and the results are not useful. An improvement is to collect some data on a cohort of hospitalized patients, either prospectively or retrospectively, and then identify those who suffered from a HAI. Patients not exposed to HAI are then matched to the patients who are exposed to HAI using factors thought likely to extend length of stay and cost. The idea is that exposed and unexposed patients are similar in terms of their risk factors, except for the presence of infection. The difference in the cost outcomes is then attributed to infection. These are often mistakenly called case-control studies, and a better description is a matched cohort study [85].

A crude or unmatched comparison between the groups would overstate the extra length of stay because the unexposed and exposed groups will differ for risk factors for increased length of stay. This is sometimes known as "bias from omitted variables." To counter this problem, the analyst can use matching to make the exposed patients as similar as possible to the unexposed controls. For each patient identified as exposed (with HAI) within the cohort, one, two or sometimes more unexposed patients are identified, which carry the same risk factors for length of stay. For example, patients may be matched on age, primary diagnosis, and/or APACHE II score. The effect of these risk factors on length of stay is now the same for both the exposed and unexposed patients. Any differences in length of stay can no longer be due to these risk factors. This gives a clearer picture of the relationship between HAI and length of stay.

Matching variables must be chosen carefully. An important limitation is that no estimate can be made of how much each matching variable contributes to length of

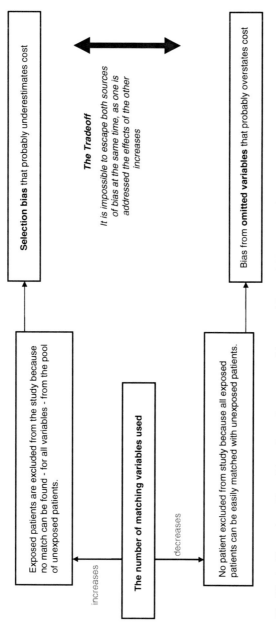

Fig. 27 An illustration of how bias arises when more and less matching variable are used in matched cohort studies

stay. There is no way of seeing the variables that are important. Therefore, there should be good existing evidence that the matching variables chosen represent true confounders between the relationship between HAI and length of stay. Residual bias will still be present in the estimate as not all confounders will be known or used for matching.

Another important problem with this method is that unexposed controls become harder to find as the number of matching variables increases. The result is that exposed patients, for whom no match can be found, are excluded from the study, and this induces another problem called "selection bias." Exposed patients are selected out of the study, because they cannot be matched with an unexposed control. Analysts, therefore, face the tradeoff illustrated in Fig. 27. Given the size of most data sets in this field of research, the maximum number of matching variables that can be used before selection bias becomes a problem is around 5–8. This journal articles shows the problems of matching studies for HAI and length of stay [86]. Both the design approaches, concurrent attribution, and matching studies have some problems.

6.3.2   Statistical Approaches

There are advantages to using statistical approaches to assess the relationship between infection and extra length of stay. Data on a cohort of hospitalized patients are used and instead of matching, and so attempting to control for differences between patients who are exposed and unexposed to HAI at the design stage, differences are controlled at the statistical analysis stage. The practice of building and evaluating statistical models can become complex but the basic idea is quite simple. Katz [87] provides a nice introduction to multivariable statistical analysis; he defines the basic approach as follows….

> Multivariable analysis is a statistical tool for determining the unique contributions of various factors to a single event or outcome. For example, numerous factors are associated with the development of coronary heart disease, including smoking, obesity, sedentary lifestyle, diabetes, elevated cholesterol level, and hypertension. These factors are called risk factors, independent variables, or explanatory variables. Multivariable analysis allows us to determine the independent contribution of each of these risk factors to the development of coronary heart disease (called the outcome, the dependent variable, or the response variable).

To interpret this definition for the example of HAI we see that "length of stay" is the outcome variable and the presence of HAI is one of the independent or explanatory factors associated with this outcome. A statistical model is illustrated in Fig. 28.

The dependent variable is the length of stay observed among the patients in the data set. The analyst believes this varies with age, comorbid conditions, whether or not they suffered an adverse event, had surgery, or most, important, whether they acquired an infection. These data in Table 10 support this theory. The residual error

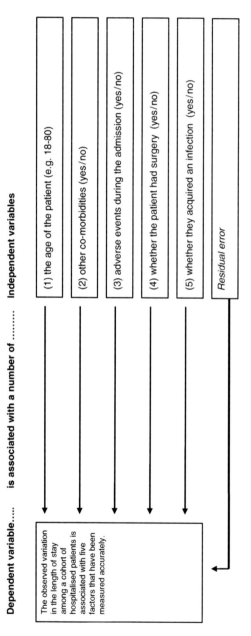

Fig. 28 A statistical model with length of hospital stay as the outcome variable

Dependent variable.....   **is associated with a number of ....**   **Independent variables**

The observed variation in the length of stay among a cohort of hospitalised patients is associated with five factors that have been measured accurately.

(1) the age of the patient (e.g. 18-80)

(2) other co-morbidities (yes/no)

(3) adverse events during the admission (yes/no)

(4) whether the patient had surgery (yes/no)

(5) whether they acquired an infection (yes/no)

Residual error

is a term included in these models to account for other variation in length of stay, not described by the independent variables measured. Models like this are designed to predict the independent effect of the explanatory factors on the outcome. The effects of the other explanatory factors have been controlled by the statistical procedure.

The advantages of this method are that all patients can be included in the statistical model and this completely avoids the problem of selection bias illustrated by Fig. 27. There is the opportunity to include a comprehensive set of explanatory terms on the right hand side of the model. Remember, matched cohort studies were restricted to 5–8 matching variables; otherwise, exposed cases were selected out. Statistical models can include many more variables, but variables should only be included if there is a good understanding of why they will explain cost outcomes like length of stay. Building statistical models gets round the problems of matching studies and can be regarded as a more appropriate research tool for addressing the problem of estimating extra length of stay.

There are challenges that users of statistical models must overcome. First is that the outcome variable, length of stay, is generally nonnormally distributed. An important prerequisite of multivariable statistical models is that the outcome variable follows a normal distribution. An example of a normal distribution is illustrated in Fig. 29. This shows that the average and most likely value for lengths of hospital stay among a cohort is approximately 5 days, and that the chances of having a longer or shorter stay are quite similar.

Unfortunately, length of stay data does not look like this. The information included in Fig. 30 is closer to how length of stay data are distributed.

This shows that most patients have a stay around 5 or 6 days but some patients stay for a long time, in this example up to 50 days. This problem of skewed data pose problems for analysts using statistical models, but a competent statistician will overcome them.

The second challenge is that, while long stays are quite rare, the longer the stay the higher the chance of infection. There are more likely to be patients with infection lurking somewhere in that long tail of the distribution. They may have hospital stays of 20, 30, or 40 days. This violates another prerequisite of statistical analyses that the independent variables or the explanatory variables on the right hand side of the model should be truly independent. In this case, we see that while HAI is likely to predict length of stay, length of stay is also likely to predict HAI, and so HAI is no longer an independent variable [88]. It is said to be "endogenously determined" and this violates another of the prerequisites for statistical models.

A solution to this issue is to account for the timing of events and so each day of the patients stay is classified as an infected day or noninfected day. More complex statistical methods, which are beyond the scope of this book, are used to account for the timing of the infection [89]. Incorporating the time of the onset of infection is potentially valuable if the objective is to estimate by how much the infection

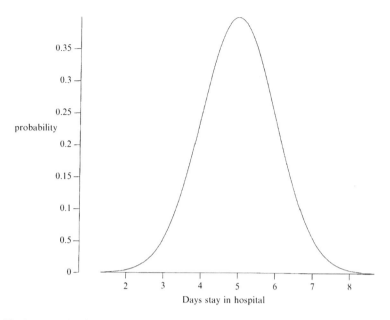

Fig. 29 An example of normally distributed data

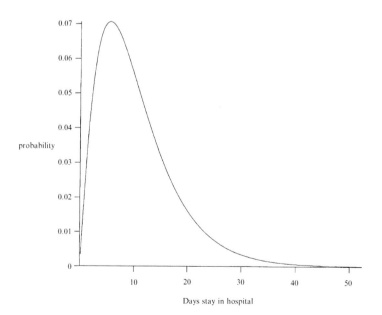

Fig. 30 An example of skewed data

prolonged stay [89, 90]. Stefan Harbarth and Matt Samore discuss these problems in more detail [85].

A third challenge is more practical in nature. HAI are, in comparison to many diseases, relatively rare events. Any dataset on which extensive modeling is to be carried out must be large. The resources required to obtain large datasets can be prohibitive, particularly if prospective data collection is to be carried out. Use of routine data from either a single source or multiple databases can still be resource intensive as it is unlikely to be clean and may require substantial work to ensure the quality and integrity of the data. These reasons help explain why there are fewer examples of this method of estimating the excess length of stay and cost, when compared with matching studies, in the published literature.

Rather than expect you to undertake complex statistical analyses, this section will allow you to be more critical of published papers that report excess length of stay and cost due to HAI. We remain with costs in the next chapter and consider some of issues faced by those who aim to measure the costs of implementing infection control programmes.

6.4 Conclusions

The likely cost savings from preventing infections is the subject of this chapter. The costs imposed by HAI should be understood and the data interpreted correctly. In particular, we warn against using cost-accounting methods to measure economic costs. Cost accountancy is used to keep a hospital financially solvent and not inform decision making about infection control. Using cost accounting data will lead to poor economic decision making. Economic principles should be used to measure costs. The process of attributing cost, in particular excess length of stay to HAI, is quite difficult. We prefer statistical models to find associations between infection and cost outcomes rather than matching exposed patients with unexposed controls.

Chapter 7
Measuring the Cost of Implementing Infection Control Programs

Preview

- The costs of implementing infection control programs are described with case studies.
- We consider the methods used to estimate the cost of infection control programs.
- The different ways that cost data can be interpreted for decision making are reviewed.

7.1 Estimating the Costs of Infection Control Programs

The costs of infection control are embedded in many departments of a hospital. Denis Spelman suggests [91].

> *In the 21st century, the specialty of infection control requires a breadth of expertise that no sole practitioner can possess. A multidisciplinary team is needed, including infection control practitioners, a hospital epidemiologist, biostatistician, infectious diseases physician and microbiologist, as well as access to a molecular biology laboratory.*

Most hospitals have a committee that oversees infection control and makes policy. This will comprise senior managers, physicians, microbiologists, and other infection control professionals. Their time is valuable and so a cost is incurred whenever they engage in activities related to the infection control committee. There might be routine surveillance programs in place that are staffed by ward nurses, who do surveillance in addition to their patient care duties. Again, their time is valuable, and the time spent on surveillance program cannot be put toward other activities. The task of running infection-control education programs is a major one, with new nursing and medical staff requiring induction to the institution's infection control procedures. The routine diagnostics and laboratory work required for infection control is also costly. A response to an outbreak of MRSA or any other resistant organism may involve a burst of activities that include a wide range of staff, from cleaning staff to laboratory workers to press officers who keep the media updated. Again, the time that these individuals dedicate to responding to the outbreak cannot

N. Graves et al., *Economics and Preventing Healthcare Acquired Infection*,
DOI: 10.1007/978-0-387-72651-9_8, © Springer Science+Business Media, LLC 2009

be used to undertake any of their other duties and thus represents the opportunity cost of infection control.

The above shows that describing the total costs of an existing infection control infrastructure is a major task. The dedicated infection control practitioners are the visible face of infection control and the costs of employing and maintaining this service can be readily assessed. Describing the costs of providing an entire infection control infrastructure, however, is quite difficult.

Fortunately, we are interested only in the costs that change as a consequence of a decision to adopt some novel or additional infection control practice. In other words, what extra costs might be incurred because of a program? The costs of additional infection control programs are represented by the arrows in Figs. 21 and 22 (Chap. 5).

7.2 Two Case Studies for Estimating the Cost of Infection Control

Economic analyses are about assessing whether some change to how resources are allocated is a good decision or not. This is why we only focus on the changes to cost that arise from some change to existing infection control arrangements. The simplest type of change to infection control might be the introduction of a new technological device. As a case study, the costs of adopting antimicrobial coated central venous catheters to replace standard catheters for all admissions to ICU are described. As a second case study, we look at the costs of introducing a more complex infection control program. The costs of implementing a multicomponent catheter care education program are described.

7.2.1 A Case Study of the Costs of Adopting Antimicrobial Catheters

An important prerequisite to describing the cost of an intervention is that the intervention is clearly defined. In this case, the proposal is to use antimicrobial coated central venous catheters instead of a standard catheter for all ICU admissions over the next 12 months. The planned change in the physical resources used should then be identified. Existing practice might be that 1,500 patients a year use a mean of 1.4 catheters per patient, this implies that $(1,500 \times 1.4) = 2,100$ standard catheters are to be replaced by an equal number of antimicrobial catheters. The cost of implementing the changes should be assessed.

A first analysis shows standard catheters cost $20 each and the antimicrobial catheters cost $45 each, so costs will change by ($45 less $20) = $25 \times 2,100 CVCs = $52,500 for the new program.

A meeting with the manufacturers reveals a better price of $40 per antimicrobial catheter is available if the decision maker commits to purchasing all 2,100. At the time this seems sensible, as costs are saved. At this price the change in costs is ($40 less $20) = $20 \times 2,100 CVCs = $42,000. Understanding the agreement reached with the suplier of antimicrobial catheters is important for estimating the economic costs of the program. The cost analyst needs to know whether the antimicrobial catheters are a variable cost (i.e., they can be escaped) or a fixed cost (i.e., the hospital is committed to the expenditures). The implications of this are worth thinking about and one that we explore in this case study.

In this case, at $40 per catheter, the costs of the antimicrobial catheters are fixed for a period of 12 months. A review of the contract with the supplier by the hospital lawyer confirms this. We are committed to paying the entire contract value of (2,100 × $40) = $84,000. A decision not to honor the contract will lead to litigation and unplanned additional costs.

After six months of the contract term, a new director of microbiology is appointed and she worries about antimicrobial resistance and decides to revert back to standard catheters. There are 1,050 antimicrobial catheters to be paid for in the stock room of the ICU. The colleagues of the new microbiologists who work in neighboring hospitals share her view about resistance, and so the antimicrobial catheters are worthless in local markets. A business manager searches for a buyer and find a hospital in another part of the country prepared to pay $10 per catheter for the unused antimicrobial catheters, but the shipping costs must be incurred by the selling hospital. The changes to costs that arise from the new program are summarized in Table 11.

Table 11 The change to costs from a decision to use antimicrobial catheters

Resource used	Cost outcome	Dollar value	Comments
Initial purchase of antimicrobial catheters	Increase	$84,000	2,100 antimicrobial catheters are purchased.
Standard catheters	Saving	$21,000	1,050 standard catheters are not purchased because antimicrobial catheters are used instead for 6 months, prior to the appointment of the new microbiologist.
Lawyer's fees for review of contract for antimicrobial catheters	Increase	$10,000	Lawyers always win.
Costs of finding buyer for antimicrobial catheters	Increase	$2,000	The business manager has to hire an assistant for 2 weeks to cover their other duties while they find a buyer.
Resale of antimicrobial catheters	Saving	$10,500	The hospital in the other state is willing to pay only $10 per catheter.
Shipping costs	Increase	$1500	Medical transport service used.
Antimicrobial resistance	Saving	Unknown	The change in policy, back to standard catheters, may well have prevented resistance to antimicrobials in the future. The value of the cost savings are not known but were certainly an important factor for this program.
Total costs		$66,000	

The real economic cost of the decision to implement the novel infection control strategy is approximately $66,000 and not $42,000 as originally thought. Many of these costs could not have been predicted before the decision was made, but the life is uncertain and decision makers have to deal with this fact.

The lessons from this case study are:

- The time frame for decision making is important. This decision was made for a 12-month period and this had implications for the costs. Had the decision been reviewed month by month, then the cost outcomes would have been different.
- The contractual obligations to make expenditures are also important and define whether the costs are fixed (inescapable in the time frame of the decision) or variable (escapable).
- A better price was obtained by agreeing to sacrifice flexibility in the contract. Had $45 per catheter been agreed then the requirement to buy all 2,100 catheters would have been avoided. The costs would have been variable within the 12 month time frame, and the decision maker could have walked away from the antimicrobial catheters when the new director made their decision.
- We live in an uncertain world, and things can change quite unexpectedly.

Estimating the costs of this relatively straightforward infection control strategy was quite complicated. Next we consider how to estimate the cost of a more complex infection control program.

7.2.2   A Case Study of the Costs of a Staff Education Program

The new director of microbiology does not like antimicrobial catheters; there is not enough information on how their adoption will increase pressure for antimicrobial resistance in the future. She has achieved reductions in infection rates in other hospitals by using education and performance feedback strategies for ICU staff and chooses to implement a similar program. It will be based around education and adopting optimal catheter insertion and management practices. The intervention will be tested for 12 months and comprises the following:

- 2 days education for all ICU staff to cover theoretical and practice aspects of preventing catheter-related blood stream infections.
- A switch to chlorhexidine as the preferred skin antisepsis prior to catheter insertion.
- Monitoring to ensure the subclavian insertion site is used where possible and that catheters are removed as soon as clinically possible.
- Performance feedback on these measures will be provided to the ICU staff by infection control professionals.

The resources to be used for this intervention are summarized in Table 12, alongside a description of the contractual obligation for the cost, the price to be paid for the resources, and total costs.

Table 12   Resources to be used for education and performance feedback program

Resource	Number of units	Cost per unit	Total	Contractual obligation
External company to provide infection control training[a]	1 training program	$10,000	$10,000	To complete 2 days training per week for an 8-week period. This is sufficient to train all ICU staff.
Agency nursing	160 h	$75	$12,000	They are remunerated for each hour they work in the ICU. The role is to provide cover while the regular ICU personnel attend the education program.
Locum physicians	40 h	$400	$16,000	
Alternate skin disinfection solution	3 batches of 50 bottles	$1,500	$4,500	These are purchased in batches of 50 bottles, three times a year.
New infection control nurse[a]	1 day/week for 12 months	$10,000	$10,000	The new infection control nurse and program administrator are offered job security for 12 months.
Admin. support[a]	0.1 full time equivalent	$5,000	$5,000	
Total			$57,500	

[a]These expenditures are fixed for the 12-month duration of the program

The total costs of the program are $57,500. Some of the costs are variable and can be escaped immediately such as the agency nursing and the locum doctors. The costs of the second and third batches of skin disinfection solution can also be avoided. The remaining costs are fixed and cannot be avoided within the 12 month time frame. We have followed the same steps as before to estimate these costs:

1. Define the novel program or intervention
2. Identify the change in resources from the new program
3. Identify the price of the extra resources
4. Analyze the contractual obligations to the expenditures (i.e., define fixed and variable costs)

7.3   Analyzing Costs, Inputs, and Outputs

The costs described in Table 12 can be thought of as the ingredients or inputs to a new process (i.e., the new infection control program). These inputs are combined together to produce something tangible and valuable (i.e., infections avoided). To understand better the costs of achieving these benefits, it is useful to consider the relationship between inputs and outputs, and how these unfold over the lifetime of the program. The purpose is to see when costs are incurred and how they relate to benefits produced. These data in Fig. 31 illustrate the inputs and the dollar cost incurred, the timing and frequency of these costs, and how they relate to the benefits of the program, the infections prevented.

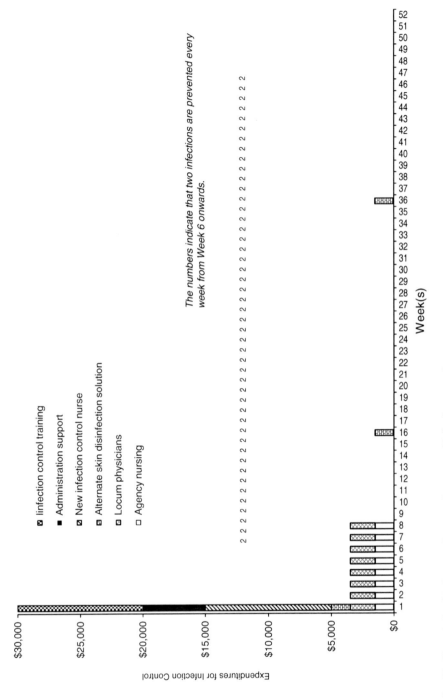

Fig. 31   The relationship between inputs and outputs of infection control

Most of the costs are incurred in week 1 when the contracts are agreed with the company providing the infection control training, the first batch of skin disinfection solution is purchased, and the infection control nurse and administration officer sign contracts. Fees for the agency nurses and locum doctors are incurred in week one, and then for the next seven weeks. After week eight, very little cost is incurred, only the batches of skin disinfectant solution at week 16 and then again at week 36. An accountant might plot these costs in terms of when the expenditures are actually made, and so the costs of the infection control nurse and administrator might appear to be spread evenly over the 52 weeks, but we are economists and are interested in what will happen if something changes. If the program was cancelled at week 4, then all the fixed costs (see Table 12) would have been incurred and are inescapable. Whether we could recoup any of these costs by trading the resources in second hand markets is another question, and one we would only seek to answer if the program was actually cancelled. For this case study, we will assume that the program runs its entire 12 month course.

The numbers plotted on the graph in Fig. 31 show that the program will prevent 2 infections per week after the run in period up to week 6. This continues over the 12 months of the program. This estimate of 2 infections per week emerged from a careful review of the epidemiological literature (see Chap. 5 on measuring the effectiveness of infection control).

The cumulative infections prevented by the new program are plotted on Fig. 32 as the thin dashed line. Figure 32 also shows the costs of the program, reported in two different ways: cumulative total costs (thick solid line) and average costs (thick dashed line). If you wish to recreate these graphs yourself, the data used to plot Fig. 31 and 32 are included in an appendix.

Plotting cumulative costs is useful as we can see when expenditures occur. These data show that a cost of $30,000 is incurred in week 1. Costs accumulate rapidly until week 8 when they are $54,500 and remain fairly stable for the remainder of the program. They do step up again twice, once at week 16 and again at week 36. Because we have retained information on the timing of these costs, we can use this data to calculate the incremental costs for the program. As we shall see, incremental costs are far more useful for making decisions than average costs.

7.3.1   Incremental Costs

Incremental costs are the amount that costs change for a given change in output. An example is the change in costs arising for another 20 infections prevented. Marginal cost is the change in cost for a one unit change in output, the change in cost from preventing one more infection. Using the data from Fig. 32, we can measure the incremental costs of this infection control program.

Week 6 is when the first two infections are prevented. At this point time costs of $47,500 have been incurred. The incremental cost of preventing these first two infections is therefore $47,500. The incremental cost of preventing the next two

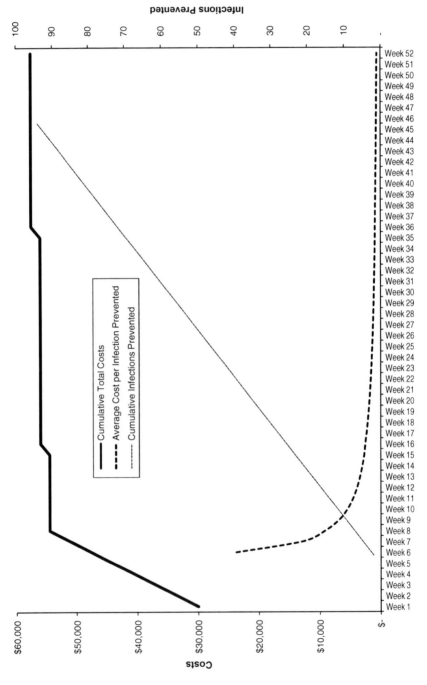

Fig. 32 Summary of cost and benefits of new infection control program

infections is $3,500 (i.e., total costs have increased from $47,500 to $51,000 between week 6 and 7). The incremental cost of preventing the next two is $3,500 ($54,500 less $51,000). After this point, costs only increase another $3,000 in total, and a further 88 infections are prevented. The upfront investments are clearly paying off as the program gathers momentum. The bulk of the cost is incurred preventing the first few infections, after that, further costs increases are minimal yet many infections are prevented.

7.3.2   Average Costs

The average cost per infection prevented is total cost divided by total infections prevented, at any given point in time. The average cost per infection prevented at week 6 is $47,500 divided by the two infections prevented = $23,750. The average costs data included in Fig. 32 show a steep decline for average cost as the program rolls out. This is because the fixed costs incurred early in the program are being spread across an increasing number of infections prevented. At week 33, the average cost per infection prevented is $1,000 ($56,000 divided by 56 infections prevented) and by the end of the program the average cost per infection prevented is $612. Estimates of cost – based on average cost – are always a function of the denominator, in this case the number of infections prevented. If this program was continued for another 2 years with only minimal changes to total costs then average cost might be driven very low, say less than $100 per infection prevented.

7.3.3   Cost Data and Decision Making

You may be wondering why we are picking costs apart in such a painstaking way. The answer is that cost estimates like these are often used for decision making to answer questions such as whether the program is an efficient investment of resources or whether it should be implemented in a new hospital. Average costs are often reported in papers and other publications, and then misinterpreted. As we have shown, average costs are determined by how long the program has been running, or put another way the scale of the program. If we were to publish these data, we might state that the cost per infection prevented was $612. This is true, but conditional on the fact that the program was run for a whole year and was successful over that year. If the program was abandoned at week 8, then $54,500 would be been spent and only 6 infections prevented, at an average cost of $9,083 per infection. Quite different conclusions would be drawn by decision makers about this program, based on these two estimates.

Further problems will arise when simple "back of the envelope" calculations are made about the changes to total costs (ΔC) from this infection control program. If some other literature showed a case of infection increased cost by $5,000, an advocate for infection control might be tempted to make the argument that savings of

$5,000 less $612 = $4,388 per infection could be achieved via the implementation of this program.

Using estimates generated in one setting, to make decisions about implementing this program in another is potentially misleading. First, it assumes that the estimate of $5,000 per infection is accurate. As we discussed in Chap. 6, estimating the cost of infection is not straightforward. Second, it assumes that the new hospital will follow exactly the same processes as the original program, and encounter exactly the same prices, market conditions, and negotiate the same contracts. Third, it assumes that the program will work on the same scale of inputs and outputs. In a setting where infection rates are much lower the absolute number of infections that will be prevented will also be lower; if this is true the program may cost the same to implement but the returns will be less.

Costing is not always straightforward. An average cost is an accessible but potentially misleading statistic. For the reasons already discussed, marginal costs, which give an indication of the relative timing of the inputs and outputs of the program, are preferred. The characteristics of every novel infection control program are going to be different, and these should be considered for all costing exercises. Poor costing methods will lead to erroneous conclusions, and if these are plotted on the cost-effectiveness plane and used for decision making, then poor decisions will result.

7.4　Capital Costs

The costs of capital items are often important for infection control. We finish this chapter with some notes for dealing with capital costs. Some infection control programs require a capital investment, and by this we mean a physical asset that will have some specialized purpose and will last for some time into the future. Examples might be the installation of a computer system that monitors hand washing activity among healthcare workers or the refurbishment of training rooms for the purposes of infection control education. The economist would be interested in looking at the obligation to the capital asset and how valuable it might be in some alternative use. If the hand washing monitoring system were leased for a short period of time, say 6 months, then we remain flexible in the decision as we can walk away from further expenditures after 6 months. Alternatively, we can commit for a five-year term and are obliged to incur costs for that period. The price will almost certainly drop if we make a long-term commitment. In this case, the stakes are high because the asset is highly specialized and has minimal value in alternative use. If we commit for 5 years, then decide the system is not worthwhile then there is nothing else we can do with it, and we still have to incur the costs. These costs are known as sunk costs, and are less desirable than resources that are fixed costs, which may have value in some other use. The decision to refurbish rooms for infection control education is less risky. Although we cannot avoid the expenditures, the asset can be redeployed for other purposes that have a value. If we decide we no longer wish to use it for the original purpose, then we have the potential to generate a revenue stream (and so offset our costs) by renting the space to other divisions in the hospital or even the open market. This asset is less specialized and so should have a value in alternative uses. It might be considered a fixed rather than a sunk cost.

These issues aside a practical approach to costing capital outlays involves two steps. The first is to consider the opportunity costs of the money tied up in the project. If we spend $100,000 on the hand washing system, then we have lost the opportunity of using that money in some other way, the interest rate charged by the bank is a reasonable proxy of the value of the costs. So if the bank pays 5% annually on savings, then the opportunity cost of the capital investment of $100,000 is $5,000 per year. The second cost is that the asset may lose value of over time. Accountants tend to write off the capital cost (i.e., depreciate) gradually over the lifetime of the asset. This is an accounting nicety that allows for prudent and careful financial planning and ensures the organization remains financially viable. The economist is more likely to consider: (i) the obligations for making expenditures, (ii) the ability to redeploy the asset for some other use that has a value. In most costing studies, the accountancy approach to depreciation is adequate but the economics of really large capital projects should be considered carefully.

7.5 Conclusions

The cost of implementing infection control should be thought through carefully. It contributes an important part of the change to total costs estimate (ΔC) that are used for decision making. Costing is not always straightforward and many factors are important. Attention should be paid to the time frame within which the infection control decision is made, whether costs can be escaped or not (i.e., whether they are fixed or can vary and indeed whether they are sunk) and how total costs, average costs, and incremental or marginal costs change over time.

Chapter 8
Preventing HAI and the Health Benefits that Result

Preview

- We define quality adjusted life years (QALYs) and show how they are calculated.
- A method to estimate the total number of QALYs gained from preventing infections is demonstrated.
- The information required to estimate QALYs is described.
- The methods for finding this information are reviewed.

8.1 Health Benefits

Changes to health benefits must be measured to assess the economics of a decision to expand infection-control. These health benefits make up the lower part of the incremental cost-effectiveness ratio (ICER) and are represented by ΔE. This was discussed first in Chap. 3 and Figs. 21 and 22 in Chap. 5 show where health benefit fit in the economic framework (look for the double headed solid horizontal arrow in the figures). The benefits of healthcare programs (ΔE) are measured in terms of quality adjusted life years (QALYs) gained for the extra-welfarist approach to economic appraisal used for this book (see Chap. 2). Reference is made to QALYs in Chaps. 2–4. We have yet to describe the methods to estimate QALYs in any detail. The goals for this chapter are to define QALYs, explain how they are measured, and review the ways of obtaining the data to estimate them.

8.2 What QALYs are and How they are Estimated

QALYs are a quantitative measure of the health gain (or health benefit) from competing programs available to healthcare decision-makers. They are composed of the duration that patients spend in a given state of health, that is, how many years they are alive in this condition, and the quality of life that they enjoy in this health state.

N. Graves et al., *Economics and Preventing Healthcare Acquired Infection*,
DOI: 10.1007/978-0-387-72651-9_9, © Springer Science + Business Media, LLC 2009

The quality of life for different health states is represented by some value between zero (i.e., dead) and 1 (i.e., healthy), and this value is called a utility score. Patients who benefit from an intervention that prevents mortality obviously represent a gain in life years. Patients who benefit from an intervention that moves them from a lesser health state to an improved health state for some period of time have enjoyed a gain in health. QALYs are designed to measure both these types of gain in one metric.

Graves et al. [9] present an example of how QALYs can be used to describe the gain in health from preventing surgical site infections following total hip replacement, and we examine the three scenarios they describe:

Scenario one – Patient with no infection. The patient never has infection related complications.

Scenario Two – Patient with a non-fatal infection. The patient has an infection that is non-fatal and they survive.

Scenario Three – Patient with a fatal infection. The patient gets an infection that causes, or interacts with other factors to cause their death.

For their example, they assume all patients receive a new hip at the same time. The health benefits that accumulate under the three scenarios are presented in terms of QALYs. To calculate these benefits, the value of the health state and the amount of time spent in that health state must be known for each scenario. Some data to describe this are included in Table 13.

All patients receive a new hip in January 2008.

Scenario one – Patient with no infection. Having received their new hip, the patient recuperates during the first quarter of that year, during which time they occupy a health state which is valued at 0.5. Remember that this number is the utility score for the health state and takes a value in the range including zero and 1. A utility score of 0.5 implies that a patient in this recuperation health state enjoys around half the quality of life enjoyed by a completely healthy individual. By April 2008, the patient's quality of life has improved and their health state or utility is valued at 0.9. They now only feel moderate discomfort from the new hip. They remain in this health state until the end of 2015. By the start of 2016 the patient is elderly and frail and their health deteriorates; the value of their quality of life is now only 0.6. They die in early 2017.

We can summarise both the life expectancy and quality of life for this patient using the QALY method. Since the new hip this patient has lived for nine years, but these years must be weighted for quality/utility in order to calculate the total number of QALYs associated with this scenario. The health state occupied for the 3 months (i.e., 0.25 years) after their surgery was valued at 0.5 and so $(0.25*0.5) = 0.125$ QALYs were accrued. The next 0.75 years (i.e, April to end of December 2008) were spent in a health state valued at 0.9 and so $(0.75*0.9) = 0.675$ QALYs were accrued. Between 2009 and 2015 (i.e., 7 years) their health state was valued at 0.9 and so $(7*0.9) = 6.3$ QALYs were accrued. In 2016 their health state was valued at 0.6 and so $(1* 0.6) = 0.6$ QALYs were accrued. Over the nine years of life this patient accrued a total of $(0.125 + 0.675 + 6.3 + 0.6) = 7.7$ QALYs.

Scenario Two – Patient with a non-fatal infection. The patient acquires an infection but makes a full recovery. This patient is very sick between January to March 2008 and they occupy a health state with a utility weight of 0.3. Between April and June 2008 things continue to go wrong and the patient acquires a secondary blood stream infection. During this time they occupy a health state valued at 0.2. By July 2008, the patient has made a full recovery and so from this point onwards, follows the same profile of health outcomes as the patient in the "Patient with no infection" scenario. The number of QALYs under this scenario can be estimated from the data in Table 13 by following the same method as the

Table 13 The hypothetical duration and value of the health states occupied by patients after total hip replacement (three possible scenarios)

Time	Scenario one Patient with no infection			Scenario two Patient with a non-fatal infection			Scenario three Patient with a fatal infection		
	Alive	Utility Score	QALYs	Alive	Utility Score	QALYs	Alive	Utility Score	QALYs
Jan-Mar 2008	Yes	0.5	0.125	Yes	0.3	0.075	Yes	0.3	0.075
Apr-Jun 2008	Yes	0.9	0.225	Yes	0.2	0.05	Yes	0.2	0.05
Jul-Sept 2008	Yes	0.9	0.225	Yes	0.9	0.225	No	0	0
Oct-Dec 2008	Yes	0.9	0.225	Yes	0.9	0.225	No	0	0
2009	Yes	0.9	0.9	Yes	0.9	0.9	No	0	0
2010	Yes	0.9	0.9	Yes	0.9	0.9	No	0	0
2011	Yes	0.9	0.9	Yes	0.9	0.9	No	0	0
2012	Yes	0.9	0.9	Yes	0.9	0.9	No	0	0
2013	Yes	0.9	0.9	Yes	0.9	0.9	No	0	0
2014	Yes	0.9	0.9	Yes	0.9	0.9	No	0	0
2015	Yes	0.9	0.9	Yes	0.9	0.9	No	0	0
2016	Yes	0.6	0.6	Yes	0.6	0.6	No	0	0
2017	No	0	0	No	0	0	No	0	0
Total QALYs			**7.7**			**7.475**			**0.125**

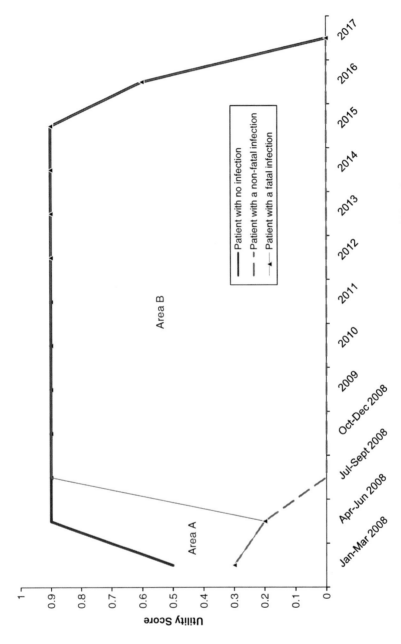

Fig. 33 The health outcomes, measured by QALYs, of three scenarios for patients undergoing total hip replacement

previous example. The total QALY gain for the nine years following hip replacement is (0.25*0.3) + (0.25*0.2) + (0.5*0.9) + (7*0.9) + (1* 0.6) = 7.475.

Scenario Three – Patient with a fatal infection. In this scenario, the patient acquires an infection and dies as a result. This patient follows the same profile for the first two quarters of the previous scenario but then dies as a consequence of the infection. The total QALYs gained are (0.25*0.3) + (0.25*0.2) = 0.125.

These data are graphed in Fig. 33. The utility score (i.e., value of the health state) is marked on the vertical axis and time is marked on the horizontal axis. The areas under the lines for each scenario approximate the total number of QALYs accumulated. Both infection scenarios result in fewer QALYs than the no infection scenario. Infections, therefore, result in a loss of health benefits as measured by QALYs. Effective infection control will avoid these infections, thereby gaining health benefits and this is what makes up ΔE.

The quantity of health benefits, measured in QALYs, for an individual patient that arise from preventing a "nonfatal infection" is indicated by the area marked with an "A." This represents the difference between the number of QALYS generated under scenario one minus the number generated under the scenario two (7.7 – 7.475 = 0.225). The size of the health benefits that arise from preventing a "fatal infection" is indicated by the areas marked "A + B" and again represent the difference between the QALYs generated in scenario one and scenario three (7.7 – 0.125 = 7.575).

Infection control programs are rarely designed for just a single patient. This method can be used to describe a cohort of patients using average utility scores. Consider a cohort of 10,000 patients who have a new hip. There will be a baseline risk of infection among the cohort under existing practice and a reduction of risk if a decision were made to expand infection-control. The baseline infection rate is 3%. The case fatality proportion among those with infection, due to infection, is 10%. If a decision were made to expand infection-control, then the infection rate is reduced to 2.2%. The proportion of these patients who die as a result of infection remains at 10%.

To analyse the health benefits achieved from an expanded infection control program, we first predict the number of infections we would expect to observe under existing practice. We then predict the number we would expect to see under then the expanded infection-control alternative. The differences between the two programs are 80, fewer infections of which 8 are fatal and are presented in Table 14.

Table 14 The number of uninfected and infected patients for existing practices vs. an expanded infection-control alternative

	Patients with no infection (a)	Total infections (b)	Fatal (c)	Nonfatal (d)
Existing practice	9,700	300 (or 3% of cohort)	30 (10% of total infected)	270 (90% of total infected))
Expanded infection control	9,780	220 (or 2.2% of cohort)	22 (10% of total infected)	198 (90% of total infected)
Difference	80	−80	−8	−72

Notes: total patients in cohort = 10,000 = (a) + (b); (b) = (c) + (d)

Rather than calculating QALYs for an individual patient, we calculate the QALYs accumulated by our entire cohort under existing practice and then for the expanded program. The difference represents the health benefits of the expanded infection control program (in QALYs) for the entire cohort. To calculate the QALY outcomes for the whole cohort under each type of infection control, we multiply the individual QALY outcomes for each scenario (Table 13) by the number of individuals in the cohort who experience each scenario (Table 14). The QALY outcomes for existing infection control practices are:

- Uninfected (9,700 × 7.7 QALYs) = 74,690 QALYs
- Fatal Infections (30 × 0.0125 QALYs) = 3.75 QALYs
- Nonfatal Infections (270 × 7.475 QALYs) = 2,018.25 QALYs

The QALY outcomes for the expanded infection control program are:

- Uninfected (9,780 × 7.7 QALYs) = 75,306
- Fatal Infections (22 × 0.0125 QALYs) = 2.75
- Nonfatal Infections (198 × 7.475 QALYs) = 1,480.05

The results are summarized in Table 15.

Table 15 The health benefits of the expanded infection control program in QALYs

	QALYs			
	Patients with no infection	Fatal infections	Nonfatal infections	Total QALYS
Existing practices	74,690	3.75	2,018.25	76,712
Expanded infection control	75,306	2.75	1,480.05	76,788.80
Differences	616	−1.00	−538.20	76.80

The overall change in health benefits (i.e., ΔE) from a decision to adopt the expanded program is the difference in total QALYs achieved relative to the QALYs that would be accumulated under existing practice. You can see in Table 15 that under the expanded program the now larger uninfected group contributes more QALYs to the total (i.e., 616 more QALYs), and the now smaller infected groups contribute fewer QALYs to the total (i.e., the sum of −1 and −538.2). The total change in QALYs or ΔE that results from the new expanded infection control program is a gain of 76.80 QALYs.

The QALY outcomes for the entire cohort under "Existing Practices" and the "Expanded Infection Control" alternative are expressed over time in Table 16. Because these QALY benefits accrue over time then they must be discounted to a net present value. After rounding up, we see the difference in QALY outcomes is 77 undiscounted QALYs but when a discount rate of 3% is used to adjust for our time preference for benefits, the value of the QALY benefits falls to 70. See Panel 6 for a description of how to discount future benefits and costs.

Table 16 The QALY outcomes for the cohort under "Existing Practices" and the "Expanded Infection Control" alternative over time (discounted values in brackets)

Time	Existing practices	Expanded infection control	Difference
Jan-Mar 2008	1,235.00 (1,235.00)	1,239.00 (1,239.00)	4.00 (4.00)
Apr-Jun 2008	2,197.50 (2,197.50)	2,211.50 (2,211.50)	14.00 (14.00)
Jul-Sept 2008	2,243.25 (2,243.25)	2,245.05 (2,245.05)	1.80 (1.80)
Oct-Dec 2008	2,243.25 (2,243.25)	2,245.05 (2,245.05)	1.80 (1.80)
2009	8,973.00 (8,711.65)	8,980.20 (8,718.64)	7.20 (6.99)
2010	8,973.00 (8,457.91)	8,980.20 (8,464.70)	7.20 (6.79)
2011	8,973.00 (8,211.57)	8,980.20 (8,218.16)	7.20 (6.59)
2012	8,973.00 (7,972.39)	8,980.20 (7,978.79)	7.20 (6.40)
2013	8,973.00 (7,740.19)	8,980.20 (7,746.40)	7.20 (6.21)
2014	8,973.00 (7,514.75)	8,980.20 (7,520.78)	7.20 (6.03)
2015	8,973.00 (7,295.87)	8,980.20 (7,301.72)	7.20 (5.85)
2016	5,982.00 (4,722.25)	5,986.80 (4,726.04)	4.80 (3.79)
Total QALYs	76,712.00 (68,545.57)	76,788.80 (68,615.82)	77 (70)

Panel 6   Discounting future benefits (and costs)

Discounting is easy. If a is the value to be discounted, b is the annual discount rate, and c is the number of years in the future that the benefit is incurred then the discounted value can be calculated using this formula,

$$\frac{a}{(1+b)^c}$$

For example, our starting year is 2008 and we wish to discount the 5,982 QALYs gained from existing practices that arise in 2016. We simply substitute the 5,982 for a, 3% (i.e., 0.03) for b and 8 (years into the future) for c,

$$\boxed{\frac{5,982}{(1+0.03)^8} = 4,722.25 \text{QALYs}}$$

Both costs and benefits that arise in future time periods should be discounted.

It is clear that multiple pieces of information are required to estimate the health benefits of an infection control program in QALYs.

Multiple pieces of information are required to estimate the health benefits of an infection control program with QALYs. First, we need to know how effective interventions might be in reducing risks, and methods for synthesizing this information were described in Chapter 5. Second, we need to know the effect of HAI on the risks of death. Third, we need to know about the nature of the health states occupied by individuals with any HAI, the time spent in those health states and the methods for finding utility scores to describe the value of the health states. These last two items – mortality risk and finding then valuing relevant health states – are the subject of the next section.

8.3   Information Required to Estimate QALYs

8.3.1   The Risk of Death due to Infection

The mortality that results as a consequence of HAI is a key parameter in any decision model about infection control. The data in Fig. 33 show that health benefits – measured in QALY gains – from preventing a "fatal" infection are great. It follows that if many lives are saved from infection control, then the number of QALYs gained from a decision to choose that infection control program will be great.

Consider a novel infection control program that causes costs to change by $500,000 (i.e., ΔC) and health benefits to change by 50 QALYs (i.e., ΔE). The ICER is $10,000 per QALY, and this represents good value for money to decision makers. The program will likely be adopted. Say the 50 QALYs arose from a modeling study that used some dubious estimate of the relationship between infection and death and a more careful subsequent analysis revealed that many patients would have died anyway and the infection merely hastened their demise. The revised number of QALYs gained might be only 5. The ICER is now $100,000 per QALY and decision makers would likely choose some other use of their scarce resources.

Our point is that the mortality attributable to (i.e., caused by) infection should be estimated as accurately as possible. It is rare that infection will unambiguously end someone life, like a gun shot wound or car crash. More often infection will interact with other factors, such as age and comorbid conditions, to hasten death. Infection control can, therefore, be thought of as averting a death, or, just slowing progress toward an inevitable death. This distinction is important and good epidemiological methods are required to disentangle the independent effect of infection on mortality risk.

Because the impact of HAI on patient mortality is such a key question, there is a substantial amount of literature available on this topic. An informed reader will interpret this information carefully. There are many similarities between the processes of attributing extra length of stay to HAI and attributing risk of death to HAI. Studies that try to quantify the magnitude of either of these outcomes are vulnerable to bias and confounding. The review in Sect. 6.3 of the different study designs used to estimate by how long infection extends stay in hospital is also relevant to this question about whether infection impacts on death risk.

Many estimates of the mortality attributable to HAI come from small, poorly designed studies. Despite this, some general trends emerge from the literature. The larger and more rigorous studies, which control for multiple potential confounders as part of the analysis, produce smaller estimates of the mortality attributable to HAI when compared with the crude comparisons. Any study attempting to provide convincing estimates of attributable mortality needs to consider controlling for the confounding effects of patient mix, risk factors, and length of stay. Estimates of the mortality resulting from ventilator associated pneumonia and bloodstream infection are generally higher than estimates produced for surgical site or urinary tract infection. Precise definitions of the HAI under investigation are important as broad categories may hide differing risks. Catheter-related bloodstream infections are thought to have a smaller effect on the risk of mortality than primary bloodstream infections and a deep tissue surgical site infection will have a greater attributable mortality than a superficial infection.

The diversity of estimates makes quantifying how each type of HAI affects patient risk of dying difficult. Some data suggests that the impact of certain types of HAI is negligible [92]. Others studies provide convincing evidence that HAI contributes heavily to risk of dying [93–95]. Part of the problem is simply down to numbers. In comparison to the number of deaths from cardiovascular diseases, the number of patients who die with a HAI is relatively small. This makes it difficult to recruit enough individuals into a study to disentangle this complex relationship between infection and mortality risk [47]. When selecting evidence on which to base a decision, the tools for assessing study quality described in Sect. 5.2.2 can be helpful in identifying which estimates are robust. Also the concepts related to study design covered in Sect. 6.3 will be useful.

8.3.2 The Nature of the Health States and the Methods for Finding Utility Scores that Describe Them

HAI causes pain and discomfort to patients. It can be relatively short-lived, like a simple urinary tract infection, or it can be prolonged and serious such as an infection of a new hip prostheses. Some infections can lead to long-term quality of life losses such as blood stream infections that cause multiple organ failure. If QALYs are used to measure the health benefits of preventing HAI, then in all cases it is important to estimate the value of the relevant health states. There are two steps to achieving this. The first is to describe the health state and the second is to assign a value between zero and one, with zero equal to the worst possible health state (or dead) and one equal feeling good.

8.3.2.1 Description of Health State

Each HAI-related health state could be described individually. For example, a urinary tract infection could be described as a "painful, uncomfortable, burning sensation, always wanting to pass urine but unable to do so," a superficial surgical site infection could be described as "tenderness around the wound and pain when the inflamed area is touched." As there are so many different types of HAI with different causes and manifestations, it would be very time consuming and costly to describe each one. To avoid this, analysts use generic questionnaires that ask about multiple attributes of health and can be used to define a wide range of possible health conditions. Brazier et al. provide a good review of these tools and their usefulness for economic evaluation [96].

One generic tool that is used for economic evaluation is the EQ-5D. This instrument can be used to value a wide range of health conditions. It is called a multiattribute utility scale because it provides a single score (i.e., a utility score on a scale between zero and one) based on participant responses to questions about five dimensions of their health. The five dimensions are:

- Mobility
- Self-care
- Usual activities
- Pain/discomfort
- Anxiety/depression.

Each has three levels of response:

- No problems = 1
- Some/moderate problems = 2
- Extreme problems = 3.

The EQ-5D is illustrated in Fig. 34.

By combining the level of response (i.e., 1, 2, or 3) for each dimension of health, a unique health state is defined. An individual who chooses level 1 for all dimensions of health (i.e., 11111) will be in a good health state with no major problems. In contrast, someone who chooses level 3 for all dimensions of health (i.e., 33333) will be in the worst health state. The SF-36 specifies 243 individual health states including 11111 and 33333. It only takes about 90 seconds to complete and can be administered as a postal survey or over the phone. The respondent is usually a participant who has the health condition for which the utility score is being derived, but it can also be completed by an informed third party, who answers on behalf of a participant who may be incapacitated. The Website for the EQ-5D is http://www. euroqol.org/. There exist other tools designed to achieve the same outcome such as the AQoL and the SF-6D. John Braziers and colleagues review provides a thorough overview of them all [96].

8.3.2.2   Valuation of the Health State

There are three popular approaches to valuing health states, regardless of whether they are described individually or defined using a generic multiattribute utility scale such as the EQ-5D. A classic paper on this was authored by George Torrance [97], and the examples included in this chapter emerge from this work. The three approaches are:

By placing a tick in one box in each group below, please indicate which statements best describe your own health state today.

Mobility

☐ I have no problems in walking about
☐ I have some problems in walking about
☐ I am confined to bed

Self-Care

☐ I have no problems with self-care
☐ I have some problems washing or dressing myself
☐ I am unable to wash or dress myself

Usual Activities *(e.g. work, study, housework, family or leisure activities)*

☐ I have no problems with performing my usual activities
☐ I have some problems with performing my usual activities
☐ I am unable to perform my usual activities

Pain/Discomfort

☐ I have no pain or discomfort
☐ I have moderate pain or discomfort
☐ I have extreme pain or discomfort

Anxiety/Depression

☐ I am not anxious or depressed
☐ I am moderately anxious or depressed
☐ I am extremely anxious or depressed

To help people say how good or bad a health state is, we have drawn a scale (rather like a thermometer) on which the best state you can imagine is marked 100 and the worst state you can imagine is marked 0.

We would like you to indicate on this scale how good or bad your own health is today, in your opinion. Please do this by drawing a line from the box below to whichever point on the scale indicates how good or bad your health state is today.

Your own health state today

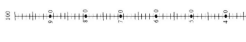

Best imaginable health state — 100

Worst imaginable health state — 0

Fig. 34 The EQ-5D standardized instrument to measure health outcome

first, marking a point on a 'Visual Analogue Scale'
second, answering 'Standard Gamble' questions
third, answering 'Time Trade Off' questions.

All three approaches have the same objective of valuing a predefined health state. Which of these three competing approaches is best is debated by health economists.

A visual analogue scale is often represented as a ruler or thermometer with equal intervals marked and defined end points, one of which is the worst outcome and the other the best. All health states lie somewhere between the extremes. The EQ-5Q includes a VAS (see Fig. 34) that can be used by researchers to value health states. Participants are asked to find a point on the scale between zero and 100, for the health state described. This process is easy for the subjects as they are not required to choose between health states when they make a valuation, they simply mark the line. The remaining two methods of "Time Trade Off" and "Standard Gamble" require subjects to make a choice.

The Standard Gamble method asks the participant to choose between two competing alternatives. We assume they currently occupy the health state – that we define as i – to be valued. Alternative 1 is to remain in health state i for t years, and then die. Alternative 2 represents a gamble on some hypothetical treatment that if they accept, will either return the participant to the best imaginable health state for t years, or cause them to die immediately. Participants are presented with the probability of winning the gamble (between 0 and 1) and being returned to perfect health. The level of probability at which they accept the gamble (Alternative 2) over the certainty of t years in the current health state (Alternative 1) is the valuation of the health state.

A participant who switches from Alternative 1 to Alternative 2, when the probability of winning the gamble (i.e., best imaginable health state) is 0.7, values state i at 0.7. The process is illustrated in Fig. 35.

The Time Trade Off method also asks the subject to choose between two alternatives. Alternative 1 is for the individual to spend the rest of their life in the health state to be valued, say t years. Alternative 2 is to spend some time less than t years, say x years, in the best imaginable health state they then die. The time in state x is then varied until the individual cannot choose between the two alternatives. At this point, the value of the health state is x/t. For example, if the subject will accept five years of good health as compensation for ten years in the health state to be valued, the worse health state, then the valuation is $5/10 = 0.5$. This is illustrated graphically in Fig. 36.

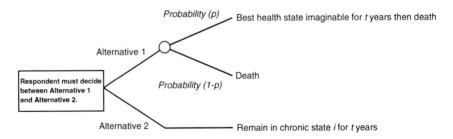

Fig. 35 Standard gamble approach to valuing health benefits

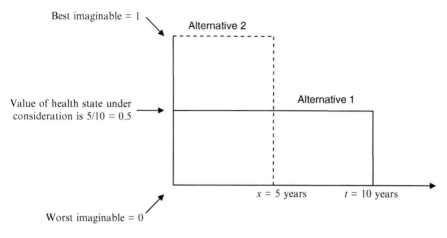

Fig. 36   The time trade off method for valuing health states

In practice, researchers prefer the choice-based methods of time trade off and standard gamble. Visual Analogue Scales are easier to use but do not force the subjects to choose between health states. Because choice is central to economics, some argue that visual analogue scales are less sound than time trade off or standard gamble questions [96].

If health states are described individually (e.g., our description of a urinary tract infection), then one of these valuation methods must be used to assign a utility weight to that health state. If, however, the EQ-5D is used to survey people with UTI, then generic valuations made by other research groups for the health states comprised by the EQ-5D can be used. A number of research groups have undertaken valuation exercises to assign a utility weight to each of these 243 predefined health states described by the EQ-5D. The complete value sets for the 243 health states that were produced by each of the research groups are available from the developers of the EQ-5D. This can simplify the process considerably. For example, we administer the EQ-5D to patients with a urinary tract infection. Hypothetically, they return scores on this instrument of 11221, indicating no problems with mobility, self care, and anxiety/depression but moderate pain/discomfort and disruption to usual activities. We can now look up the health state of 11221 in the value set from the United States, which gives us a utility weight for urinary tract infection. The value sets available are summarized in Table 17: as you can see they are estimated for different countries. Researchers prefer to use value sets produced in a country with characteristics most similar to their own context. This is because norms around tolerance to pain or the effect or loss of functional ability may vary across settings.

An alternative to using multiattribute tools such as the EQ-5D is to map data collected using the generic health surveys, SF-36 and SF-12, onto preference-based utility scores. The process by which SF-36 and SF-12 data are revalued using preference elicitation methods are described by Brazier and colleagues [25, 26]. They

Table 17   Value sets produced as part of the EuroQol Group enterprise

Country	Number of subjects that took part in the valuation exercise	Valuation method
Belgium	548	Visual Analogue Scales
Denmark	1,179	Visual Analogue Scales
Denmark	1,332	Time Trade Off
Europe	6,870	Visual Analogue Scales
Finland	928	Visual Analogue Scales
Germany	339	Visual Analogue Scales
Germany	339	Time Trade Off
Japan	543	Time Trade Off
New Zealand	919	Visual Analogue Scales
Netherlands	298	Time Trade Off
Slovenia	370	Visual Analogue Scales
Spain	294	Visual Analogue Scales
Spain	975	Time Trade Off
UK	3,395	Visual Analogue Scales
UK	3,395	Time Trade Off
US	3,773	Time Trade Off
Zimbabwe	2,384	Time Trade Off

Source: EuroQol group (http://www.euroqol.org/)

developed the SF-6D tool, which provides preference-based valuations for both standard SF-36 and SF-12 data. The SF-6D is copyrighted but the only requirement is that users register their projects with the research team.

8.4   Conclusions

The health benefits that arise from investing in more infection control are just as important as the changes to cost outcomes. Without understanding health benefits, economic appraisal cannot be done. They are measured by changes to quality and quantity of life: these are captured with quality adjusted life years, QALYs. To calculate the difference in QALYs from some infection control program, it is important to quantify risks of infection under different infection control programs and the risk of death due to HAI. We also need to understand the nature of the health states occupied by individuals, the time spent in those health states, and the methods for finding utility scores that value the health states.

Chapter 9
Dissecting a Published Economic Appraisal

Preview

- The processes undertaken for a real economic appraisal of an infection control alternative is described and the complexities of the tasks are revealed.
- Each task is documented so the reader can see what was done, where the task was difficult, and what caveats were built in.
- A description of how the findings might be used to inform decision making is also included.
- Most of this book has used hypothetical examples to convey ideas and theory. This chapter is a description of a real decision problem for the infection control community.

9.1 Economic Evaluation in the Infection Control Literature

The rationale for an economic model has been covered in earlier chapters of this book. The concepts used to construct and evaluate a decision model were discussed in Chaps. 3 and 4. The types of data on costs and health outcomes that are required to inform an evaluation were covered in Chaps. 6–8. The information in these chapters provides a grounding in the methodological steps involved in economic evaluation and you may like to refer back to them while reading this chapter. The concepts introduced in previous chapters should not be used as a black and white checklist against which models are held up to pass or fail. They should be viewed as a set of tools to be used by those undertaking an evaluation.

The processes of undertaking a real evaluation may be more complex than these appear on paper. The time and resources required to complete the evaluation are likely to be scarce. Each evaluation will present different challenges. Some evaluations will have more data available or more complex disease processes than others. Sometimes good data may have already been collected and for other evaluations some prospective data collection may be required.

In this chapter, we show how we evaluated the economics of using antimicrobial-coated central venous (A-CVC) catheters to prevent catheter-related bloodstream infection. This real-world application shows the complexity of the processes and the collaborations required to produce a rigorous study. We do not attempt to

N. Graves et al., *Economics and Preventing Healthcare Acquired Infection*,
DOI: 10.1007/978-0-387-72651-9_10, © Springer Science + Business Media, LLC 2009

prescribe a one-size fits-all recipe for conducting an evaluation, but aim to point out some of the issues faced by those developing models and raise awareness of possible approaches to dealing with them. This chapter will be useful for those both critiquing evaluations and constructing their own economic decision models.

9.2 Case Study of a Decision to Adopt Antimicrobial Central Venous Catheters

Central venous catheters coated or impregnated with antimicrobial agents have been available since the early 1990s. These catheters have been the subject of clinical trials in a variety of patient populations. A number of systematic reviews of this evidence have been undertaken which indicate that they are effective at reducing the rate of catheter-related bloodstream infection in intensive care unit and general ward patients [98–101].

The cost is roughly three times that of uncoated catheters. Given the number of devices used for patient care, a decision to switch to antimicrobial-coated devices would represent a significant change to costs. If the catheters are effective there will be cost-savings by avoiding infections. A decision to adopt this technology requires consideration of the changes to health outcomes and economic costs. This point is made in the 2002 Centers for Disease Control and Prevention Guidelines for the Prevention of Intravascular Catheter-Related Infections [102]:

> "The decision to use chlorhexidine/silver sulfadiazine or minocycline/rifampin impregnated catheters should be based on the need to enhance prevention of CR-BSI after standard procedures have been implemented (e.g., educating personnel, using maximal sterile barrier precautions, and using 2% chlorhexidine skin antisepsis) and then balanced against the concern for emergence of resistant pathogens and the cost of implementing this strategy."

The best way to approach an economic evaluation of this technology is via a decision analytic model (see our discussion in Sect. 4.1). The main reason is that several different types of A-CVC are commercially available and each varies in terms of price and effectiveness. There is no trial that compares all types of A-CVC directly yet the decision maker is interested in comparing the costs and health benefits of all types, side by side. This can only be achieved with a decision model. Many of the A-CVC trials were not powered to detect a difference in rates of CR-BSI and instead used the surrogate outcome of catheter colonization. Even fewer were large enough to report other important outcomes such as mortality attributable to infection. A model-based evaluation allows evidence from diverse sources (i.e., from outside the clinical trials) to be included for these important parameters.

9.3 Structuring the Evaluation

An expert panel of infection control practitioners, infectious disease clinicians, and ICU physicians was convened. Their role was to review the scope of the research, the assumptions, and the design of the evaluation. A primary task was to find the clinical scenario, patient population, timeframe, and interventions to be studied. Our panel worked within the healthcare system of Queensland, Australia and were interested in the efficiency of a decision to adopt these catheters within the public health system. The group recommended evaluating whether A-CVCs should be used routinely within the adult intensive care unit (ICU) setting. The rationale was that this was a controlled environment, good data existed on ICU activities, and outcomes and patients in ICU experience a higher rate of complications than other wards.

The main outcome was the incremental cost per quality-adjusted life year gained. All costs and QALY benefits that occurred in future years were discounted at a rate of 3% in line with recommendations [103, 104].

The structure of the model emerged from discussions with the panel of experts. Relevant events and likely patient prognoses were identified and these are described in Table 18 Each event was incorporated because it has clinical or economic importance. The events of CR-BSI and mortality represent important outcomes in terms of health and economic costs. Some clinical events, that would not affect the economic appraisal, such colonization of the catheter and adverse reactions to the A-CVCs, were discussed but excluded from the model. Adding them would increase complexity and not provide insights to the economic decision.

The remaining events were organized in the model displayed in Fig. 37.

Each outcome needed to be defined. Death is unambiguous but for others, such as catheter-related bloodstream infection, there are multiple definitions. The Centers for Disease Control and Prevention clinical definition of CR-BSI was used. This was chosen over a surveillance definition because its use was more common in the literature from which we would be sourcing many of the data.

The interventions chosen for comparison were the A-CVCs commercially available in the Australian setting:

- Minocycline and rifampicin coated (MR)
- Silver, platinum and carbon impregnated (SPC)
- Chlorhexidine and silver sulfadiazine internally & externally coated (CH/SSD int/ext)
- Chlorhexidine and silver sulfadiazine externally coated (CH/SSD ext)

These four catheter types are compared to one another and a baseline comparator, an uncoated catheter. All would be assumed to be polyurethane, triple-lumen, and available in standard dimensions. The decision to be evaluated is illustrated in Fig. 38. Remind yourself of what the square node, first discussed in Chap. 4, represents.

Table 18 Events that reflect the prognoses of an ICU patient in the decision model

Event	Included?
Catheterization	All patients assumed catheterized
Colonization	No
Catheter-related bloodstream infection	Yes
Adverse reaction to A-CVC	No
Catheter removal	Yes
Discharged alive	Yes
Mortality	Yes

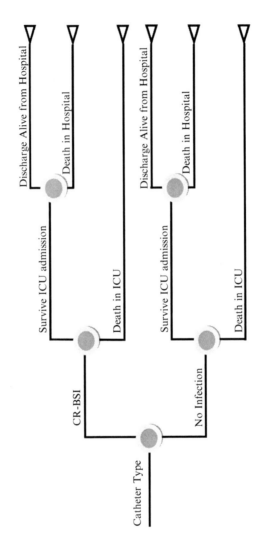

Fig. 37 Structure of the decision model, chance events branches

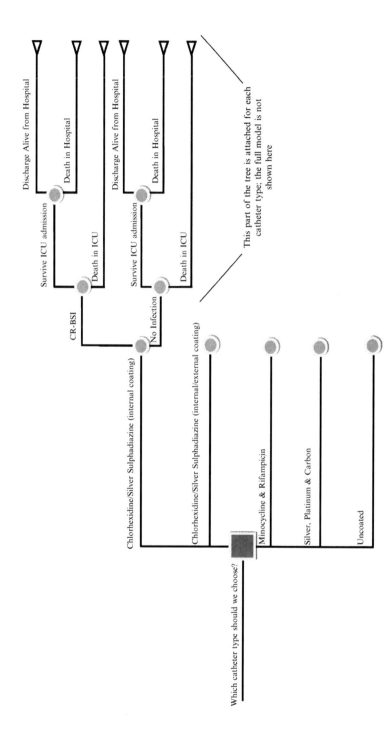

Fig. 38 Structure of the decision model, initial decision (square) node

9.4   Evidence Required for the Evaluation

Many data items are required to inform this decision model. Estimates are needed of costs, disease rates, utility weights, and mortality risk. The best way to measure effectiveness is by a randomized controlled trial; however, data for some of the other estimates might be of higher quality and usefulness if sourced from individual databases, registries, and government bodies. The goal is to find the best data for the job at hand. The data required to inform the parameters for this model can be broken down into several main types:

- Epidemiological parameters
- Effectiveness of the A-CVCs
- Cost outcomes
- Health outcomes

The data used for the evaluation are given in Table 19. Some of the advantages and disadvantages of each data source are included.

We did not have sufficient resources to collect primary data to inform model parameters. Instead published estimates were used for most parameters. The exception was costs of consumable items used as a result of infection. This information came from within the Australian public healthcare system. One challenge was that there were multiple estimates for parameters in the model. In each instance, we

Table 19 Estimates used to parameterize the A-CVC model

Parameters		Baseline estimate	Source	Notes on data source
Infection-related events				
Probability of CR-BSI		2.5%	Database	Representative, required confidentiality agreement
RR Mortality (CR-BSI)		1.41	[105]	Most rigorous and accurate studies
Extra days in ICU		2.4 days	[106]	identified but still quality low,
Extra days on hospital ward		7.5 days	[106]	process of identification complex
Effectiveness A-CVCs (RR infection)				
SPC		0.54	[100]	Data are available for all types of A-
CH/SSD (ext)		0.66		CVC in this review
CH/SSD (int/ext)		0.70		
MR		0.39		
Baseline probabilities of mortality				
ICU mortality		7.7%	[107]	Easy to source, representative
Hospital mortality		3.4%	[108]	Representative of decision context,
Annual mortality postdischarge	Year 1	5%	[108]	study type (linkage) prone to error and bias
	Years 2–3	2.7%		
	Years 4–5	2.8%		
	Years 6–10	3.7%		
	Years 11–15	4.2%		
Underlying annual mortality	45–64 years	0.4%	[109]	Easy to access but takes time to request data, representative of decision context
	65–84 years	3.0%		
	85+ years	14.0%		

(continued)

Table 19 (continued)

Parameters		Baseline estimate	Source	Notes on data source
Utilities				
Utility ICU		0.66	[110]	Easy to source, elicitation methods poor, not representative
Utilities population norms	50–59 years	0.80	[111]	Representative of decision context, elicitation tool not tested in other settings therefore comparability reduced
	60–69 years	0.79		
	70–79 years	0.75		
	80+ years	0.66		
Costs, 2006 AUD				
ICU bed day		$3,021	[112]	Easy to source, may not truly repre- sent opportunity costs
Hospital bed day		$843	[113]	
Diagnostics CR-BSI		$102	Database	Representative of decision context, required confidentiality agreement, may not translate across settings

used the highest quality data available. To help judge the quality of the evidence, we used the "quality of evidence hierarchy" for economic analyses [60] combined with Braithwaite et al. [114] evidence valuation hierarchy and Harris et al. [115] review of quasiexperimental study designs. This made the process of choosing the data for the model transparent and resulted in the best information being used.

9.4.1 Epidemiological Parameters

Information on the population of catheterized patients was retrieved from publicly avail- able data contributed by 46 public tertiary referral ICUs to the Australia New Zealand Intensive Care Society [107]. This helped us generalize the results to a national context. The ICU cohort had a mean age of 60.7 years (SD = 17.2), mean APACHE II score 16 (SD = 8) and 55% were emergency admissions. We assumed that half of this population would receive a CVC during their stay in ICU [116] and that these individuals would not differ in any systematic manner from those who did not require catheterization.

Rates of CR-BSI, using uncoated catheters, were calculated from routine surveillance data collected from 21 medium-to-large public hospitals in Queensland, Australia [117]. In the absence of a national surveillance system, data from a regional system was thought to be adequate. We were reassured that the estimates were quite similar to those found from other regional surveillance systems in Australia [118]. The data reported from this surveil- lance system were available as the number of infections per 1,000 catheters placed.

9.4.2 Effectiveness of Antimicrobial CVCs

A key parameter was the effectiveness of the different types of A-CVC. All had been the subject of randomized controlled trials. The results of the systematic review and meta-analysis that summarized evidence for the effectiveness of all four commercially available types of A-CVC [100] were used. This meta-analysis showed how effective the A-CVCs were relative to uncoated catheters in terms of risk ratios. The relative risk of CR-BSI, given use of each catheter type, was then applied to the baseline risk of infection observed for uncoated catheters.

9.4.3   Costs

Information on the costs were organized into those items for which a price could be directly observed (i.e., something akin to a market price; you could return to Chap. 1 to read about markets and the price system), and, items for which the opportunity cost had to be imputed. Costs will not transfer easily between settings as market prices for healthcare resources will vary (e.g., the cost of employing a nurse in the US may be quite different from the cost of employing a nurse in Thailand) and the valuations of opportunity costs, such as a bed day released depend on the structure of the healthcare system. We therefore sought estimates from the literature which related specifically to the Australian public health system.

The directly observed costs included consumable items such as diagnostic tests, antibiotics to treat infection and of course the catheters. These are variable costs. The use of these resources was measured and cost values attached using the purchasing records and contracts held in the hospital or healthcare system databases. Costs for each of the antimicrobial-coated catheters were sourced from purchasing agreements within the health system. This reflects that when negotiating large contracts the price per unit may change (see Sect. 7.2.1). Where contracts did not exist, the local representative for the company responsible for distribution of the catheter was contacted for an estimated supply price based on the volume and duration of an anticipated contract.

The other main cost parameter was the bed days lost to infection. These account for most of the fixed costs of running a hospital. Because they are fixed expenditures for them will not change, regardless of rates of infection. The bed days can, however, be used in another way and so have some opportunity cost. The first step to measuring this opportunity cost is to gather information on the number of extra days of hospitalization in both the ICU and general ward, which result from infection. Multiple estimates for this parameter were found in the literature; our search retrieved 19 articles. Each was assessed using Braithwaite and colleagues tool that was designed to judge the quality of evidence used for decision analytic modeling [114]. As several useful estimates were available, preference was given to the study with the greatest similarity in healthcare setting and patient mix to that used in the evaluation [106].

The second step was to assign an economic value to a bed day. The value for an ICU bed day came from a detailed costing study conducted within an Australian ICU [119] and the value for a general bed day came from data on government spending for Australian public hospital services [113]. These estimates were derived from a cost accounting process and are likely to reflect the average cost (see Chap. 6 again). The preferred alternative would be to elicit the decision-makers' willingness to pay for the marginal bed day, but this was beyond the scope of our resources. This would be a nice study to do. Nevertheless we believed the estimates would approximate the marginal value of a bed day, and, alternate values were explored by sensitivity analyses.

Some cost estimates referred to an earlier time period. In order to account for inflation we updated these costs to 2006 prices using the Bureau of Labor Statistics Consumer Price Index (http://www.bls.gov/cpi), which provides inflation ratios for costs. This process is discussed in Panel 7.

An intervention which cost $5,000 to implement five years ago will cost more to implement today as the prices of the resources and staff salaries will have risen. This is due to inflation. So it would be incorrect to use the estimate of $5,000 directly in your evaluation. To get around this problem we can update costs to reflect current prices using inflation ratios.

The Bureau of Labor Statistics Consumer Price Index provides data on how much a fixed quantity of medical care costs each year relative to what it cost in 1982-4 and presents this in units called index points. The 1982-84 baseline is set at 100 index points. The index points required each year for the period 1990 – 2006 are shown in the table. You can see that 336.2 index points are needed in 2006 to access the same bundle of medical care.

We can calculate the inflation ratio for each earlier year relative to the current year (here 2006) by dividing the index points in the current year by those from the earlier year. From here the process of updating costs is straightforward.

Our estimate of the value of an ICU bed day came from a study conducted in 2003 that estimated the cost to be $2,670. To update this to 2006 values we simply multiply the estimate by

Year	Index points	Inflation ratio
1990	162.8	2.065111
1991	177	1.899435
1992	190.1	1.768543
1993	201.4	1.669315
1994	211	1.593365
1995	220.5	1.524717
1996	228.2	1.473269
1997	234.6	1.433078
1998	242.1	1.388682
1999	250.6	1.34158
2000	260.8	1.28911
2001	272.8	1.232405
2002	285.6	1.177171
2003	297.1	1.131606
2004	310.1	1.084166
2005	323.2	1.040223
2006	336.2	1

the appropriate inflation ratio: $2,670 x 1.131606 = $3,021 in 2006 prices

Panel 7 Updating costs to 2006 prices

9.4.4 Health Outcomes

Infection rates and the quality-adjusted life years for each catheter type were tracked by the model. Infection rates are calculated within the model by applying the reduction in risk of CR-BSI achieved by each A-CVC to the baseline rate of infection. QALYs are comprised of data on patient's life expectancy and the utility of the health states which they occupy while alive. The different methods available to estimate these weights are the subject of Chap. 8.

To calculate the life expectancy of patients, a baseline estimate of mortality for this population was produced. Risk of ICU mortality came from the Australian and New Zealand Intensive Care Society (ANZICS) national database that was also used to define our patient population [107]. Annual mortality rates for 15 years post-ICU discharge were taken from a data linkage study [108] that followed over 10,000 Australian ICU patients. It was the largest study available with the lengthiest follow up period. Subsequent life expectancy was based on Australian Institute of Health and Welfare published age-specific mortality rates [109].

We identified and selected information on the attributable mortality by reviewing the quality of each study. This excess risk of death was then applied to patients within the model who developed CR-BSI [105]. After discussion with our panel of experts we assumed no elevated risk of mortality following infection post-discharge.

In order to calculate QALYs, we assigned preference-based utility weights to the time that patients spent in the ICU and for 6 months post-discharge. This information was available from the published literature. Fourteen studies reported utility weights for the ICU patients. Values were used from the study [110] with participant demographics similar to our cohort and which used an instrument (i.e., the EQ-5D) shown to predict weights similar to the Australian Quality of Life (AQoL) instrument that was used to derive the population quality of life norms [120]. Life expectancy for those surviving beyond the first 6 months post-ICU was adjusted using AQoL utility [111].

Originally we thought to assign a utility weight specifically to those patients who developed a CR-BSI. However, on researching this parameter it became clear that no estimates were currently available in the literature specifically for this health state. Previous evaluations of sepsis [121] had used utility weights for acute respiratory distress syndrome on the basis that this condition was of comparable disease severity. Discussion with our expert panel indicated they believed this to add unnecessary uncertainty to the model. Therefore, we decided to be conservative in our evaluation and no further decrement was attributed to CR-BSI.

9.5 Evaluating the Decision

Having developed our model using an appropriate structure and identified and incorporated the evidence we were in a position to evaluate the decision. The expected costs and health benefits from choosing each type of A-CVC are summarized in Table 20.

Table 20 Costs and QALYs of uncoated vs. antimicrobial CVCs

	Incremental costs (AUD $, 2006)	Incremental infections (rate per 1,000 catheter days)	Incremental QALYs	ICER
Uncoated	–	–	–	Dominated
CH/SSD (ext)	−97,603	−1.89	0.65	Dominated
CH/SSD (int/ext)	−54,935	−1.67	0.57	Dominated
SPC	−125,929	−2.57	0.88	Dominated
MR	−138,102	−3.42	1.17	Cost-saving

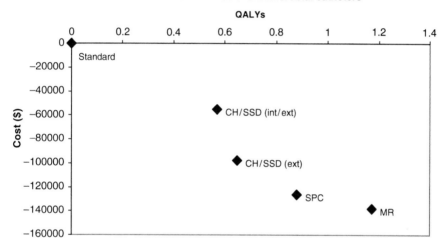

Fig. 39 Cost and QALYs of uncoated vs. antimicrobial CVCs, graphed

All the A-CVCs are cost saving relative to the use of uncoated catheters. They achieve greater health benefits and generate cost-savings within the healthcare system. This represents a "win win" for decision makers. This outcome is described in the "Introduction" chapter and by Fig. 21 in Chap. 5. A graphical representation of our result is plotted on the cost-effectiveness plane in Fig. 39. The MR catheters represent the optimal choice. The full version of this paper is published in Critical Care Medicine (2009:13;2) by Kate Halton and colleagues.

9.6   Handling Uncertainty in the Decision

All decisions are made in the presence of uncertainty. Failure to recognize the presence of uncertainty, and explore the impact it may have, can at best reduce the relevance of an evaluation, and at worst render it useless for real-world decision making. We have explored this issue in a journal article about the decision to adopt A-CVCs [59].

The robustness or stability of this decision in the face of uncertainty is important. Testing the model with uncertainties can build confidence in the conclusions drawn from the model. If a decision is stable despite the uncertainty, strong conclusions can be drawn about the cost-effectiveness of the intervention. If a decision is unstable to uncertainty this provides valuable information to the decision maker about where uncertainty is concentrated.

An exploration of the effect of uncertainty – like any statistical analysis – should have a clear plan. The sources of uncertainty in the decision to adopt the use of A-CVCs included parameter uncertainty, data quality, model structure, and the generalizability of the evaluation. We discuss each of these and consider how we might explore the impact of this uncertainty on our conclusions.

9.6.1   Parameter Uncertainty

Parameter uncertainty is derived from random error in the estimates used to inform model parameters. Evaluations must make some attempt to capture the information provided by the confidence intervals and standard errors rather than just point estimates. Probabilistic sensitivity analysis and cost-effectiveness acceptability curves, introduced in Chap. 4, achieve this. All parameters in this model were characterized as probability distributions except costs which were assumed known in this decision-making context. The model was run 10,000 times drawing different values for each parameter from within the bounds of their respective confidence intervals.

The results of the probabilistic sensitivity analysis are shown by the cost-effectiveness acceptability curve in Fig. 40. The decision is considered over a range of

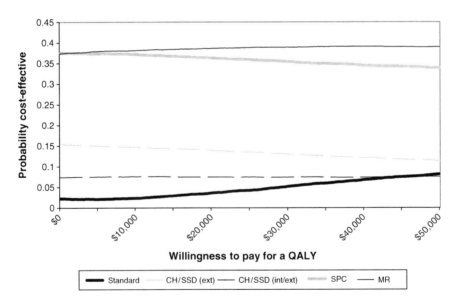

Fig. 40 Results of the probabilistic sensitivity analysis presented as a cost-effectiveness acceptability curve

ceiling ratio thresholds for QALYs between 0and $50,000 (see Sect. 3.3 for a discussion of ceiling ratios). The data in Fig. 40 show the probability that one type of catheter is cost-effective, for a range of ceiling ratios. The decision is therefore dependent on the decision-makers' willingness to pay for QALYs. The catheter type with the highest probability of being cost-effective over almost the entire range of thresholds ($3,800–$50,000) is the MR catheter (i.e., the thin black line). Below a ceiling ratio of $3,800 per QALY, the SPC catheter is preferred.

There is a lot of uncertainty introduced by the data to this decision. Even at a high willingness to pay threshold of $40,000 per QALY, there is a 39% chance that the MR catheter is cost-effective and a 34% chance that the best decision is an SPC catheter. A decision maker might feel uncomfortable choosing based on this result. The best way to help the decision maker is to collect additional data that allows key parameters to be estimated with improved accuracy. This will make the process of choosing less uncertain.

This analysis does, however, rule out the other catheter types. At no point across the whole range of willingness to pay thresholds do either the standard catheters (thick black line) or the CH/SSD catheter types (the black and gray dashed lines) become the optimal decision. Even taking uncertainty in the underlying data into account, the evidence suggests that standard and CH/SSD catheters are unlikely to be cost-effective compared to the other catheter types.

9.6.2   Data Quality

Everyone has heard of the phrase "garbage in, garbage out" and historically this has proved a challenge for many decision models as at best it affects the credibility of results and at worst produces misleading conclusions. In this evaluation, we looked at the source of the data included in the model and ranked each piece according to whether it was high, medium, or low quality. We used a tool developed for decision-analytic models to help judge the quality of each data source [60].

To explore the impact of data quality on our results a series of sensitivity analyses were done. The parameters based on medium- or low-quality evidence were reappraised by the expert panel. The utility estimates for ICU patients and the values per bed day in the ICU and the general ward came under scrutiny. The conclusion was not sensitive to different values for ICU patient utility. The conclusion was, however, sensitive to the economic value placed on a bed day in the ICU or general ward. This is consistent with the decision being driven by economic costs rather than health benefits. When a higher value was given for bed days the MR catheter remained the best choice. At lower values the silver, platinum, and carbon catheter was preferred. If bed days were assumed to have zero economic value, then uncoated catheters were optimal. A healthcare system with no waiting lists for hospital would attach a zero or very low value to bed days released by infection control.

This analysis shows that if the extra bed day released by preventing cases of infection can be used to treat more patients, thereby increasing revenue for the hospital, these bed days have a high economic value (i.e., opportunity cost); and the MR catheters are optimal (for a full discussion of this point, see this paper [4]). If on the other hand there is no waiting list for the ICU and no demand for extra bed days, then they hold zero economic value. Under these conditions the uncoated catheter is the best option. Although this scenario is unlikely as most countries have some kind of waiting list for their healthcare services, the provision of this information to the decision maker enables them to judge for themselves which scenario best represents conditions within their own healthcare system.

9.6.3   Generalizability

Factors such as the healthcare context, patient mix, and perspective of the evaluation need to be taken into account. In this evaluation, we made the assumption that the results of this evaluation would be valid across all public ICUs within Australian teaching hospitals due to the use of national databases and involvement with experts from a broad range of institutes and backgrounds.

The provision of this information enables the reader to judge where the similarities and dissimilarities between the setting of the evaluation and their own context lie. A factor which may hinder this transparent reporting is the word limit given by journals which restricts the volume of information that may be presented. This is not a problem unique to economic analyses and many journals now give authors the opportunity to publish appendixes containing technical information with the online version of their article.

9.7   Interpreting the Results for Decision Making

In this setting, and given a willingness to pay for QALYs of $40,000, we conclude that MR catheters are the most likely to be cost-effective when compared to the other catheter types on the market. At low willingness to pay thresholds for health benefits the SPC catheters are the most likely to be cost-effective. While it may be difficult to choose between the two types, they clearly dominate the use of standard and CH/SSD catheters across the range of willingness to pay threshold considered.

This conclusion is sensitive to the value placed on both ICU and hospital bed days. When low economic value is placed on bed days the SPC catheters become the cost-effective option even at high willingness to pay thresholds. The uncertainty in the underlying data both in terms of its precision (parameter uncertainty) and quality therefore makes choosing between the SPC and MR catheters difficult. Despite this uncertainty though there is a clear indication that either of these is preferred over the standard and CH/SSD catheters.

It is important to recognize other weaknesses in the evaluation that may undermine its usefulness for decision makers and discuss these in relation to the results of the evaluation. This example, of the decision to use A-CVCs, did not consider the potential for the MR antibiotic catheters to contribute toward increases in anti-biotic resistant organisms. This element of the decision was not included due to a lack of data. However, this is a real consideration for clinicians.

Some of the practicalities of undertaking an economic evaluation for an infec-tion control intervention have been discussed in this chapter. Before embarking on your own you should think about whether you need an economic evaluation. Some decisions will be clear cut that common sense will prevail. Switching from brand name to generic antibiotics is an example. Also, make sure evaluations do not already exist? If they do, you should undertake a careful critique of the work to identify whether you can apply the results directly to your situation.

9.8 Conclusions

The last decade has witnessed an increase in the amount of economic evidence available in the infection control literatures. This information is valuable to a number of different stakeholders within the healthcare system but it is important that only rigorous and well-conducted evidence is used for decision making. Poorly executed evaluations or ones that do not address relevant questions are not useful for decision-making.

Chapter 10
Economic Facts and the Infection Control Environment

Preview

- The rapidly changing infection control environment is described.
- The implications for hospitals and infection control professionals are reviewed.
- Some economic facts are presented and interpreted for infection control professionals working in this new environment.
- A frame work for good regulation of infection control is presented.

10.1 The Changing Infection Control Environment

The infection control environment is changing and a key driver is the rise of patient safety. Patient safety is important. Hospital patients are vulnerable to poor practices among hospital workers that may change their risk of suffering a healthcare acquired infection, or some other adverse event. An event as simple as a doctor not washing his hands prior to an examination may cause the transmission of microorganisms that colonizes the patient, leading to an infection or even contributing to their death. The epidemiology of infections among patients is reported by government-funded surveillance systems and calls are made to implement programs that reduce risk.

The preventable nature of these events has lead to the development of a National Patient Safety Foundation (http://www.npsf.org/au/) to reduce rates. Research into preventive strategies in this area has expanded rapidly. A search on the National Center for Biotechnology Information database (http://www.ncbi.nlm.nih.gov/sites/entrez) for "patient safety" found almost 6,000 published articles. A scientific journal, The Journal of Patient Safety, is dedicated to improving patient care and minimizing harm. The methods used to evaluate the efficiency of adopting programs to reduce risks are a major part of this book.

The payers of health care have traditionally been held responsible for meeting the costs of dealing with infections and other adverse events. If a patient in a US hospital gets an infection that prolongs their stay by 5 days and increases variable costs by $4,000, most of the cost would be funded to the hospital by the Centers for

N. Graves et al., *Economics and Preventing Healthcare Acquired Infection,*
DOI: 10.1007/978-0-387-72651-9_11, © Springer Science + Business Media, LLC 2009

Medicare & Medicaid Services or some organization that pools risks (i.e., community health programs, private sector health programs, health maintenance organizations, or employer-provided insurance schemes). In a system such as the United Kingdom's National Health Service, where health care is funded from general taxation and is free at the point of consumption, healthcare providers are also protected from the costs. The costs are borne by the individuals who pay insurance premiums and general taxes.

There is no economic incentive to reduce risk to those who have most control over the chance of the adverse event happening. Of course, healthcare professionals are highly trained and take pride in supplying the best care possible for their patients. However, clinical practice can be highly stressful, microorganisms evolve, new technologies emerge, the hospital environment is complex and busy, and other needs, perceived to be more urgent, can crowd out best practice. Those with most influence over risk are largely protected from the costs of that risk. Instead, the costs are distributed between the patient, their families, and the third party payers that fund healthcare services; this problem is known as moral hazard.

It might be tempting to increase accountability among healthcare workers. Imagine a scenario where a surgeon had the costs of treating surgical site infections that arose among their cases deducted from their fees. This crude approach would never be a good strategy, for many reasons, but making agents more accountable for their behaviors can be a powerful policy tool.

The US government recently gave in to that temptation and sanctioned the Centers for Medicare and Medicaid Services to withhold payments to hospitals for adverse events that were thought to be avoidable by the application of evidence-based guidelines [122]. The final list of avoidable events relating to healthcare-acquired infection included catheter-associated urinary tract infections, catheter-related blood stream infections, and surgical site infections after defined elective surgeries such as orthopedic surgery and bariatric surgery [122]. Staphylococcus aureus septicaemia, Clostridium difficile associated disease, and Legionnaires' disease were originally included, but removed from the list after negotiation with the Infectious Diseases Society of America and the Society for Healthcare Epidemiology of America. The objective of the legislation is to reduce cost and improve patient outcomes.

The legislation came into force on October 1, 2008. The result was to shift the costs of certain infections onto those who provide healthcare services, i.e., the hospitals, and protect the third party payers, i.e., CMS, from costs they cannot directly control. This is a bold move by the US government. The implications for infection control professionals in the US are profound. It is unlikely that private insurers and other health funds will not follow this lead and the trend may spread to other international settings. The regulation implies:

1. Infections are expensive.
2. Infection control is relatively cheap.
3. Investing in infection control will pay for itself and deliver health benefit.

4. Every single case of certain types of infection can be prevented.
5. It is cost-effective to prevent every single case.
6. Hospitals will have perfect information on the cost-effectiveness of all infection control programs and so will choose the best allocation of resources for infection control.

The goal for the next section of this chapter is to critique these points using the economic theory developed in the preceding chapters of this book. Economic facts will be exposed, and the way they relate to this new infection control environment will be discussed.

10.2   The Economic Facts

There are three economic facts relevant to the logic used in the CMS argument. First, most quality control activities show diminishing returns. Second, hospitals have quite distinctive cost structures. Third, there is a deficit of information about the cost-effectiveness of competing infection control programs.

10.2.1   Diminishing Returns

The first economic fact is the law of diminishing returns. The law states that over time the gains achieved from continued investment in an activity will start to decline. In other words, if you double what you put in you will not double what you get out. This logic is present in many areas of life. For example, if you are given one cup of coffee your ability to concentrate increases. A second cup of coffee does not double your powers of concentration, it just increases them slightly. A third cup of coffee may actually reduce concentration. You are getting successively less output (ability to concentrate) for your inputs (coffee).

As applied to the CMS regulation, the law of diminishing returns relies on the idea that initial reductions in the infection rate may be easier to achieve than subsequent reductions, as infections will become increasingly complex and resource intensive to prevent as the infection rate falls. A hospital administrator who employs one infection control nurse, one session of an infectious diseases physician and provides a budget for microbiology and diagnoses will achieve good infection control outcomes. By adding to these resources, say by investing in a surveillance program and a hand hygiene education program, further gains are likely. Purchasing antimicrobial-coated central lines may provide additional benefits but installing ultra clean air systems in the theaters may do little over and above the other activities to reduce infection rates. There will come a time where marginal investments for infection control add lesser amounts of marginal benefit in terms of infections avoided. The relationship between investments in infection control (inputs) and the benefits that result (outputs) are illustrated in Fig. 41.

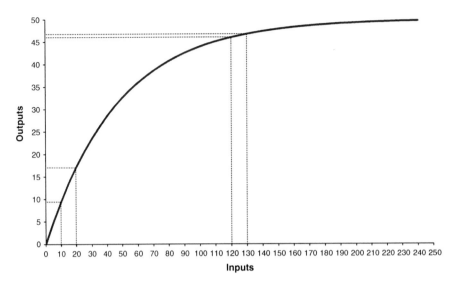

Fig. 41 Diminishing marginal returns

These data points show that increasing the inputs for an activity produces lower marginal outputs. For example, a change in inputs from 10 units to 20 units yields a change in outputs of 9.5–17 (a gain of 7.5); however, an increase from 120 units to 130 units yields a lower return of just 0.75 units of output. In the context of infection control, investments to this activity are inputs, and the reduction in infections (or increase in the number of infections prevented) is the gain in output. This concept can be shown more clearly if the data points are redrawn in a slightly different way (i.e., flipped around), but the reasoning remains the same. Look at Fig. 42.

To interpret the data we read that it is less costly to reduce rates from 20 to 15% (the cost is $64,529) than to reduce rates from 10 to 5% (the cost is $169,914). As more money flows toward infection control, the gains diminish. To reduce rates from 4 to 3%, high costs of $260, 784 are incurred. The data used to plot Fig. 42 are included in Table 21.

Diminishing marginal returns are an economic fact and one that should not be overlooked when designing regulation that affects infection control decisions. The implication of the CMS ruling is that certain HAIs should be eradicated; otherwise the hospital will have to pay the economic consequences. This might be unfair for a couple of reasons.

It might not be cost-effective to eradicate HAIs. The data in Fig. 42 and Table 21 show that the cost per infection prevented grows as we move toward zero. An economist would ask what else would be done with these resources, or, what is the opportunity cost? A good example of this is provided by Persson and colleagues [123] who undertook research on the economics of preventing infection, and so revision, among total hip replacement patients. They considered three strategies to prevent infection, use

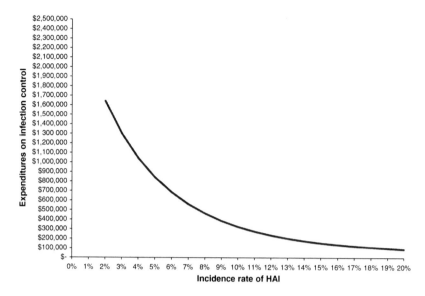

Fig. 42 Diminishing marginal returns and the costs of infection control

Table 21   Diminishing marginal returns, infection control

Expenditures on infection control	Incidence rate of HAI (%)
^	0
^	1
$1,642,939	2
$1,303,920	3
$1,c043,136	4
$841,239	5
$683,934	6
$560,602	7
$463,307	8
$386,089	9
$324,445	10
$274,953	11
$235,003	12
$202,589	13
$176,164	14
$154,530	15
$136,752	16
$122,100	17
$110,000	18
$100,000	19
$90,000	20

^Technologically feasible?

of a surgical enclosure, provision of systemic antibiotics, and gentamicin impregnated cement to secure the joint. They found diminishing returns from infection control. A decision to use all three of these strategies was the most effective, but was predicted to change costs by $314,000 in order to prevent one deep infection. They commented that the money might be deployed with greater efficiency to some other part of the healthcare system. You can think back to the discussion of MRSA screening, surgical robots, and upgraded IT systems in Chap. 1.

Another reason the CMS ruling may be unfair is that some infections are impossible to prevent and eradication is not technologically feasible. This point is made in Table 21 as no cost data are shown for rates below 2%. An "impossible zone" may exist between rates of 2% and zero (i.e., eradication), yet this is what hospitals must achieve, according to the regulator.

We suggest that when decisions are made that have implications for an entire health system, there will always be some residual risk of infection among a population of hospital patients. Some hospitals will achieve eradication and case studies have been described by Zell and Goldman [124]. Hospitals whose core business is performing elective surgeries for a generally healthy/wealthy community might be able to move toward eradication. Hospitals that care for higher risk individuals, such as those with a suppressed immune system due to chemotherapy or HIV/AIDS, for example, may be unable to prevent infection regardless of any action taken.

These arguments allow valid criticism of the CMS regulation, or any copycat regulation in another setting. The dilemma faced by hospitals is that failing to eradicate certain HAIs incurs a financial penalty. The source of the penalty is the refusal by the payers of healthcare services to meet the costs of the care required to treat the infection. Instead the hospital has to fund the shortfall from some other source. If hospitals do attempt to eradicate infections, they become exposed to this problem of diminishing returns and will likely waste scarce resources that could be better utilized for other programs. This potentially inefficient allocation of resources is a drain on the health system and should be avoided. Hospitals are caught between a rock and a hard place.

10.2.2   Cost Structures

The second economic fact pertinent to the CMS regulation is that most of the costs of running a hospital are fixed in the short run. The difference between fixed and variable costs is important and was considered in some depth by using examples in Chap. 6. The fixed costs of running a large and complex organization like a hospital cannot be easily avoided by hospital administrators. Rebecca Roberts published a paper in JAMA [75] that showed 84% of the costs of running a US hospital were fixed and these included the costs of labor, equipment, building space, and maintenance. The implication for the hospital administrator is that even if rates of infection are reduced, fixed costs will remain and they must be paid for.

The situation is awkward because revenues will fall when payers stop reimbursing the costs of infection, but the fixed cost commitments still have to be met. The only cash savings that will be made from reducing infections will be for variable costs. These are items like dressings, saline solutions, and antibiotics. These savings are likely to be relatively minor compared to the loss of revenues. There will be an initial shortfall between revenues earned and costs that must be paid.

There is of course a positive side to reducing rates of infection. The average length of stay will fall because fewer patients acquire infection. Bed days are released for alternate uses, and these alternate uses may have a positive economic value. The opportunity cost of healthcare acquired infection is therefore the value of the bed day released, in its next best use. This depends on whether marginal patients can benefit from using these bed days and whether they can find a payer willing to fund their admission. If bed days are redeployed and additional revenues flow, then these contribute to fixed costs and the hospital administrator breathes a sigh of relief. They will of course have to pay the extra variable costs of the new admissions. These arguments are presented in Chap. 6 (see Sect. 6.2.2, titled the economists view of the costs of infection) and the mechanisms that cause these change to costs have been explained, in some, detail, in a journal article [4]. Indeed, it is likely that a hospital's revenue will increase at a faster rate than their costs with new admissions, and so the average cost per patient may fall. Under this assumption, the costs of HAI are positive for the hospital. More patients treated for the same stock of fixed costs will have improved efficiency.

The payer for health care has, however, increased rather than decreased their spending. More patients are treated and average cost is likely to fall but total payer expenditures will rise. The current interpretation of cost savings by the CMS regulators appears to be simplistic and assumes that preventing a case of infection will save the hospital cash; we do not think this will happen.

If the regulator is determined to save cash expenditures in the future by reducing rates of HAI, then the only strategy to achieve this is to make hospitals smaller by reducing the size of their fixed costs. The physical size of the building will have to be reduced by employing building contractors; this will have the effect of reducing fixed overheads such as heating, lighting, and facilities maintenance. The number of staff will have to be reduced by not renewing employment contracts as they expire in the future. Capital machinery such as MRI and CT scanners will have to be sold in second-hand markets. All these things take time and so we deduce that fixed costs can only be reduced in the long run. Real cash savings can only be achieved in the long run and will result in a smaller, but more efficient hospital system.

It is important to interpret correctly how costs change with reduced infections. The positive economic costs from tolerating infections have been assumed for the hospital, and so prevention will save economic costs. Accordingly, we plot the costs of infection as increasing with incidence on Fig. 43.

This shows the cost of infection control (characterized by diminishing marginal returns) and the costs imposed on the hospital by HAIs. At rates of 20% the costs of infection are just over $2,000,000. The next step is to think about the aggregate

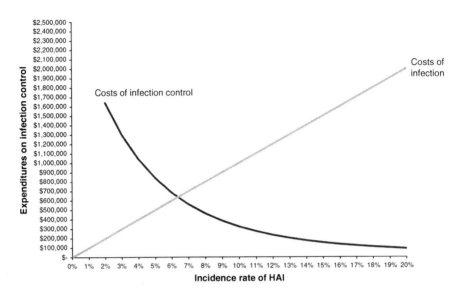

Fig. 43 The cost of infection control with diminishing marginal returns and the cost of infection

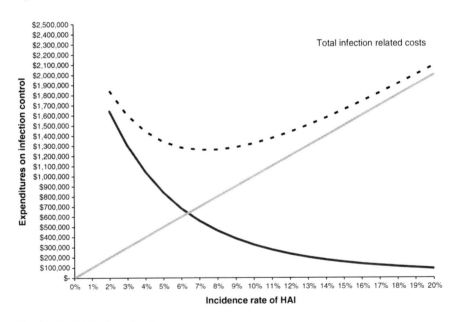

Fig. 44 Total infection related costs

costs related to infection. These arise from adding the two lines together, total infection-related costs are plotted on Fig. 44.

Regulators such as the CMS can now observe that driving rates toward zero will in fact increase costs to the hospital. Every infection rate less that 7% causes an

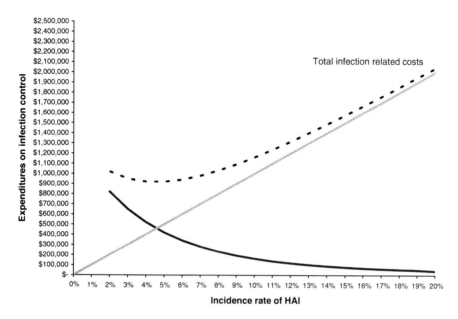

Fig. 45 Total infection related costs (now with a subsidy from the payer)

outcome where aggregate costs are higher. Regulators might not be able to sell their regulation on the grounds that it is cost saving. The hospital administrator who wishes to minimize their costs will prefer the rate of 7%. There are no economic incentives to reduce rates further, despite the attempts of the regulator. The regulator could pay the hospitals to increase infection control. This subsidy has the effect of reducing the costs of infection control to the hospital and the scenario is illustrated in Fig. 45. The best rate for hospitals will now be just under 5% rather than 7%.

10.2.3   Lack of Good Information

The third economic fact is that there is a lack of good information on the costs and cost-effectiveness of preventing healthcare-acquired infection. Evidence-based guidelines, such as those published by the Centers for Disease Control, only consider clinical effectiveness and do not provide any data on cost outcomes or cost-effectiveness. The graphs plotted in Fig. 43–45 have assumed that some data are known with certainty, in particular:

- What infections actually cost (i.e., the extra length of stay due to infection, the value of the opportunity costs of the bed days lost to infection and the variable costs used to treat the infection)
- The costs of implementing every relevant infection control strategy
- The effectiveness of every relevant infection control strategy

Without these pieces of information it is impossible to plot these graphs.

The reality for hospitals is that data on the costs of infection are scarce and potentially misleading. Some of the methodological problems arising among studies that attribute cost to HAI were described in Chap. 6. Furthermore, the information available about the cost-effectiveness of infection control is limited. Patricia Stone has published two reviews [2, 3] that show the coverage of information and its quality are both lacking. Ben Cooper [125] published a review on MRSA control strategies that showed existing studies are likely to be misleading and are characterized by threats to their validity.

The cost-effectiveness of strategies to reduce risk of catheter-associated blood stream infection has been studied more than any other type of HAI. Despite this, the authors of a review of this literature [59] concluded

> "Evidence is incomplete, and data required to inform a coherent policy are missing. The cost-effectiveness studies are characterized by a lack of transparency, short time-horizons, and narrow economic perspectives. Data quality is low for some important model parameters."

High-quality data are required on the costs and cost-effectiveness of strategies that reduce HAI. When these data are available the graphs plotted in Fig. 43–45 can be drawn for real. Until this happens, hospitals will implement infection control but will not know whether it is cost-effective or not. This can create incentives for behavior which undermines, rather than promotes, infection control within hospitals.

10.3   Incentives for Bad Behavior

The existence of these three economic facts may create incentives for some inappropriate behavior among hospitals [126].

Hospitals facing financial penalties from a failure to eradicate might mis-classify healthcare-acquired infections as community acquired, thus avoiding the financial penalty. In rare cases, patients perceived to be at very high risk of infection may be refused admission because the hospital will not want to pay for any infection that occurs. We began this book by describing the achievements of the SENIC program which indicated that prospective surveillance was an essential part of any good infection control strategy. Since then high-quality surveillance has been an important part of the infection control professionals' toolkit [127]. The incentives for transparent and valid prospective surveillance may be eroded because reporting rates of infection will reduce income for the hospital.

Physicians may be tempted to use more antibiotics as prophylaxis, or may resort to using antibiotic-coated/impregnated devices such as catheters, prostheses, or other devices. Although effective, and so attractive for decision makers in the short term, this may increase the pressure for selection of resistant organisms in the future [128] and render current antibiotics such as methicillin ineffective. The evidence for this is convincing. In 1987, two in every 100 ICU patients did not respond to methicillin, yet by 2004, more than 50 in every 100 did not respond [129]. Ramanan Laxminarayan and Gardner M. Brown look at this problem as economists [130]. They liken antibiotic effectiveness to a natural resource such as minerals, forests, or stocks of fish in the oceans. These resources are open to anyone who can acquire them and many individuals can access the benefits from the resource at the same time. They are therefore prone to overuse and will diminish rapidly if their extraction goes unchecked. This was called the Tragedy of the Commons by Garrett Hardin [131] who argued that many self-interested individuals can destroy a shared resource even when in the long term it benefits no one for this to happen.

Hospitals administrators may face pressure to cut costs inappropriately because they are down on revenue and this may even harm efforts to prevent infections. Remember, the only costs they can cut quickly are variable costs. These might include items that actually protect against infection such as hand hygiene products, cleaning services and staff education programs. In the longer term they might try to make fixed costs variable by not renewing longer term staff contracts but instead just retaining a key clinical faculty and using agency healthcare workers to cover busy periods. This working arrangement has been shown to increase rates of infection [132]. The regulators must be careful that attempts to driving rates to zero are not counterproductive.

The previous sections have been quite critical of the CMS attempts to regulate hospitals in order to improve infection outcomes. So, what do we think good regulation looks like? This question is addressed in Sect. 10.4 and summarizes much of the material covered in Chaps. 1–9.

10.4   Good Decision Making for Infection Control

To address this question we go right back to the beginning of the book and think about using scarce resources efficiently. The data plotted on Fig. 46 show some infection control decisions that are efficient and some that are not. They are marked with the letters "a" to "e."

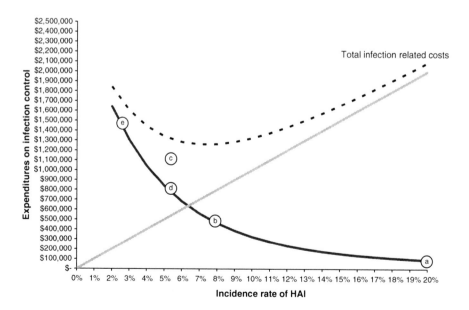

Fig. 46 Total infection related costs and the cost-effectiveness of infection control strategies

Our starting point with a high rate of infection, say 20%, is marked by "a." We observe the decision to adopt an infection control program that leads to economic outcomes marked by point "b" is better than to remain at point "a." The reason is that total costs are lower (i.e., the dashed line that shows total infection related costs falls over this range) and health benefits are higher (i.e., a lower incidence rate is achieved). This "win win" is rare in today's stressed healthcare environment. Infection control offers the opportunity to save costs while improving health outcomes and no one can argue against that. Indeed, choosing to stay at point "a" is unethical as it wastes money and harms patients at the same time. Choosing infection control that leads to economic outcomes marked by point "b" is therefore a good decision.

We would never want to remain at point "a" and so we take point "b" as a new starting point for decision making. A decision that leads to economic outcomes marked by "d" is always better than a decision that leads to outcomes marked by point "c," when compared to the new starting point of point "b." The reason is that health benefits are the same, rates of 5% are achieved with both "c" and "d," but "d" is lower cost. A decision to move to point "d" is cost-effective as compared to a decision to move toward point "c." Note that both costs and health benefits have increased by moving from point "b" to point "d." Costly infections are prevented but the savings do not compensate the costs of obtaining them. Overall costs increase but health outcomes improve for patients. The slopes of the lines that show the costs of infection and the costs of infection control provide proof. The value for money of the decision that moves us from "b" to "d" must be compared to other ways of using health care dollars to generate health benefits. If choosing "d" is better value than some other use of scarce resources then it should be adopted.

The option of moving to point "e" is also relevant for decision makers, but note that costs increase faster per unit of health benefit gained than ever before. Even if "b" to "d" was cost-effective it might be the case that "d" to "e" is not. It depends on the incremental cost per unit of health benefit gained (i.e., the incremental cost-effectiveness ratio) and whether this is below our threshold of willingness to pay for health benefits. As we have discussed, infection control is not immune from diminishing returns that affect virtually all quality improvement activities. We can see the diminishing returns arising from the steepness of the line that shows the costs of implementing infection control in the region between "d" and "e." If the ICER for "d" to "e" is above our threshold we would stop at point "d."

These data can be mapped onto something altogether more familiar, the cost-effectiveness plane. This was introduced in Chap. 3 and has been used throughout the book. All that needs to be done is for reduced incidence rates of infection to be presented in terms of quality-adjusted life years gained. Remember infections reduce quality of life and increase risk of death and preventing them will generate QALYs. Figure 47 shows the cost-effectiveness plane and economic outcomes marked by point "b" as compared to point "a." They occupy a point in Quadrant II which implies these programs should always be implemented.

Point "b" is a good decision and so now becomes the start point for any other decisions, or the new version of "existing practice." The economic outcomes of all the other programs, relative to point "b," are marked on Fig. 48.

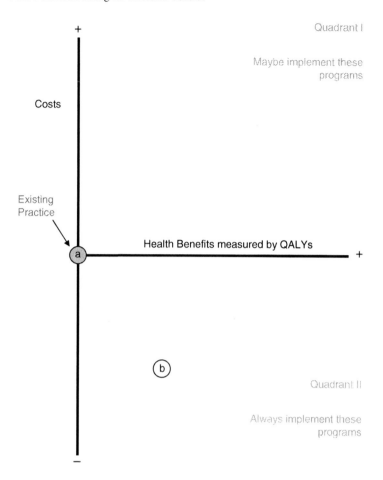

Fig. 47 The cost-effectiveness plane for policy making – mark I

Good decision making for infection control requires discarding option "c," because it achieves the same level of health benefit as option "d" for higher cost. Next the value for money of option "d" and then "e" should be assessed according to the decision-makers' willingness to pay for health benefits (see Sect. 3.3 in Chap. 3). If the cost per QALY for "d" vs. "b" falls below the threshold then it should be adopted and if the cost per QALY for "e" vs. "d" is above the threshold then it should not.

Good decision making can only emerge from good data and good data can only emerge from good research. This is what the infection control community must achieve. There are many strong research groups working on really novel methods for the evaluation of healthcare-acquired infection. Relationships between them should be encouraged and the best way for this to happen is to fund collaborative research.

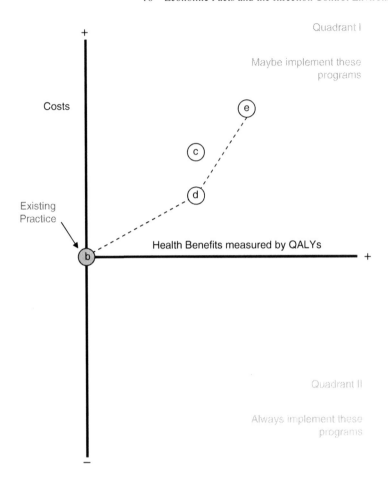

Fig. 48 The cost-effectiveness plane for policy making – mark II

10.5   Conclusions

The infection control environment is changing with the rise of patient safety and tougher regulation from those who pay for health care. These changes must be considered against the backdrop of three economic facts: diminishing returns to infection control; a high level of fixed costs among hospitals; and, a lack of good data on the costs of infection and the cost-effectiveness of infection control programs. Good decision making for infection control will only emerge from consideration of these facts and particularly requires more research and more information. There are many skilled infection control practitioners and researchers available, their efforts should be harnessed with funding and collaboration.

Appendix

Summary of the costs of and number of infections prevented by the new infection control program

	Cumulative total costs	Cumulative infections prevented	Average cost per infection prevented
Preprogram	$0	0	n/a
Week 1	$30,000	0	n/a
Week 2	$33,500	0	n/a
Week 3	$37,000	0	n/a
Week 4	$40,500	0	n/a
Week 5	$44,000	0	n/a
Week 6	$47,500	2	$23,750
Week 7	$51,000	4	$12,750
Week 8	$54,500	6	$9,083
Week 9	$54,500	8	$6,813
Week 10	$54,500	10	$5,450
Week 11	$54,500	12	$4,542
Week 12	$54,500	14	$3,893
Week 13	$54,500	16	$3,406
Week 14	$54,500	18	$3,028
Week 15	$54,500	20	$2,725
Week 16	$56,000	22	$2,545
Week 17	$56,000	24	$2,333
Week 18	$56,000	26	$2,154
Week 19	$56,000	28	$2,000
Week 20	$56,000	30	$1,867
Week 21	$56,000	32	$1,750
Week 22	$56,000	34	$1,647
Week 23	$56,000	36	$1,556
Week 24	$56,000	38	$1,474
Week 25	$56,000	40	$1,400
Week 26	$56,000	42	$1,333
Week 27	$56,000	44	$1,273
Week 28	$56,000	46	$1,217
Week 29	$56,000	48	$1,167
Week 30	$56,000	50	$1,120
Week 31	$56,000	52	$1,077
Week 32	$56,000	54	$1,037
Week 33	$56,000	56	$1,000

(continued)

Appendix (continued)

	Cumulative total costs	Cumulative infections prevented	Average cost per infection prevented
Week 34	$56,000	58	$966
Week 35	$56,000	60	$933
Week 36	$57,500	62	$927
Week 37	$57,500	64	$898
Week 38	$57,500	66	$871
Week 39	$57,500	68	$846
Week 40	$57,500	70	$821
Week 41	$57,500	72	$799
Week 42	$57,500	74	$777
Week 43	$57,500	76	$757
Week 44	$57,500	78	$737
Week 45	$57,500	80	$719
Week 46	$57,500	82	$701
Week 47	$57,500	84	$685
Week 48	$57,500	86	$669
Week 49	$57,500	88	$653
Week 50	$57,500	90	$639
Week 51	$57,500	92	$625
Week 52	$57,500	94	$612

References

1. Cohen DR, *Economic issues in inection control*. J Hosp Infect, 1984. 5 (Supplement A): 17–25.
2. Stone PW, Larson E, and Kawar LN, *A systematic audit of economic evidence linking nosocomial infections and infection control interventions*: 1990–2000. Am J Infect Control, 2002. 30: 145–52.
3. Stone PW, Braccia D, and Larson E, *Systematic review of economic analyses of health care-associated infections*. Am J Infect Control, 2005. 33(9): 501–9.
4. Graves N, *Economics and preventing hospital-acquired infection*. Emerg Infect Dis, 2004. 10(4): 561–566.
5. Clarke SKR, *Sepsis in surgical wounds with particular reference to Staphlyococcus aureus*. Br J Surg, 1957. 44: 592–596.
6. Martone WJ, et al., *Incidence and Nature of endemic and epidemic nosocomial infections, in Hospital Infections*, Bennet, JV and Brachman, PS, Editors. 1992, Little, Brown and Company: Boston. 577–596.
7. Byford S, Torgerson DJ, and Raftery J, *Cost of illness studies*. BMJ, 2000. 320: 13-35.
8. Drummond MF and Davies LF, *Evaluation of the costs and benefits of reducing hospital infection*. J Hosp Infect, 1991. 18 (Supplement 18): 85–93.
9. Graves N, Halton K, and Lairson D, *Economics and preventing hospital-acquired infection – Broadening the Perspective*. ICHE, 2007. 28(2): 178–84.
10. Haley RW, *Cost-Benefit Analysis of Infection Control Activities, in Hospital Infections*, Brachman P and Bennett J, Editors. 1998, Pippincott-Raven: Philadelphia, PA. 249–267.
11. Plowman RP, Graves N, and Roberts JA, *Hospital Acquired Infection*. 1997, Office of Health Economics; London.
12. Saint S, et al., *The role of economic evaluation in infection control*. AJIC, 2001. 29: 338–44.
13. Scott RD, Soloman SL, and McGowan JE, Applying Economic principles to Health Care. Emerg Infect Dis, 2001. 7(2): 282–285.
14. Cantril H, *The Pattern of Human Concerns*. 1965, Rutgers University Press; New Brunswick, NJ.
15. Keynes JM, *Economic Possibilities for our Grandchildren, in Essays in Persuasion*, Keynes JM, Editor. 1963, W.W. Norton & Co.: New York, NY, 358–373.
16. Samuelson P, *Economics*. 1948, McGraw-Hill, Columbus, OH.
17. Smith A, *An Inquiry into the Nature and Causes of the Wealth of Nations. Fifth edition.*, Cannan E, Editor. 1904, Methuen and Co., Ltd: London.
18. Stiglitz JE, *Economics of the Public Sector*. 1999, Norton; New York/London.
19. Harford T, *The Undercover Economist: Exposing Why the Rich Are Rich, the Poor Are Poor – and Why You Can Never Buy a Decent Used Car!* 2006, Oxford University Press: New York, NY.
20. Cookson R, *Willingness to pay methods in health care: a sceptical view*. Health Econ, 2003. 12: 891–894.
21. Arrow KJ, *Uncertainty and the welfare economics of medical care*. Am Econ Rev, 1963. 53: 941–73.

22. Williams A, *Health Economics: the cheerful face of the dismal science, in Health and Economics*, William A, Editor. 1987, Macmillan: London.
23. Maynard A and Kanavos P, *Health economics: An evolving paradigm*. Health Econ, 2000. 9: 183–190.
24. Hamp RD, Sherbourne CD, and Mazel RM, *The Rand 36 item health survey 1.0*. Health Econ, 1993. 2: 217–218.
25. Brazier J, et al., *Deriving a preference-based single index from the UK SF-36 health survey*. J Clin Epidemiol, 1998. 51(11): 1115–1128.
26. Brazier J, Roberts J, and Deverill M, *The estimation of a preference-based measure of health from the SF-36*. J Health Econ, 2002. 21: 271–292.
27. Merrer J, et al., *Complications of femoral and subclavian venous catheterization in critically ill patients – A randomized controlled trial*. JAMA, 2001. 286(6): 700–707.
28. Neuhauser D and Lewicki A, *What do we gain from the sixth stool guaiac*. N Engl J Med, 1975. 293: 226–28.
29. Klitzman B, et al., *Pressure ulcers and pressure relief surfaces*. Clin Plast Surg, 1998. 25(3): 443–50.
30. Briggs AH and O'Brien BJ, *The death of cost-minimization analysis*. Health Econ, 2001. 10(2): 179–84.
31. Sugden R and Williams A, *The principles of practical cost-benefit analysis*. 1978, Oxford; Oxford University Press.
32. Coast J, *Is economic evaluation in touch with society's health values*. BMJ, 2004. 329: 1233–1236.
33. Donaldson C, Currie G, and Mitton C, *Cost effectiveness analysis in health care: contradictions*. BMJ, 2002. 325: 891–894.
34. Klok RM and Postma MJ, *Four quadrants of the cost-effectiveness plane: some considerations on the south-west quadrant*. Expert Rev Pharmacoecon Outcomes Res, 2004. 4(6): 599–601.
35. O'Brien BJ, et al., *Is there a kink in consumers' threshold value for cost-effectiveness in health care*. Health Econ, 2002. 11(2): 175–180.
36. Torgerson DJ and Spencer A, *Marginal costs and benefits*. BMJ, 1996. 312: 35–36.
37. Weinstein M, *From cost-effectiveness ratios to resource allocation: where to draw the line?* in Valuing Health Care, Sloan FA, Editor. 1996, Cambridge University Press, New York, NY, 77–96.
38. Kanis JA, et al., *Treatment of established osteoporosis: a systematic review and cost-utility analysis*. Health Technol Assess, 2002. 6: 1–146.
39. National Institute for Clinial Excellence (UK), *Guidance on the use of computerised cognitive behavioural therapy for anxiety and depression*. Vol. NICE Technology Appraisal Guidance no.51. 2002, London.
40. Brown RE, Hutton J, and Burrell A, *Cost effectiveness of treatment options in advanced breast cancer in the UK*. PharmacoEconomics, 2001. 19: 1091–102.
41. Clegg A, et al., *Clinical and cost effectiveness of surgery for morbid obesity: a systematic review and economic evaluation*. Int J Obesity, 2003. 27: 1167–77.
42. Garber AM and Phelps CE, *Economic foundations of cost-effectiveness analysis*. J Health Econ, 1997. 16: 1–31.
43. Phelps CE and Mushlin AI, *On the (near) equivalence of cost effectiveness and cost benefit analysis*. Int J Technol Assess Health care, 1991. 7: 12–21.
44. Drummond MF and Jefferson TO, *Guidelines for authors and peer reviewers of economic submissions to the BMJ*. Br Med J, 1996. 313: 275–283.
45. Gold MR, et al., *Cost-effectiveness in Health and Medicine*. 1996, Oxford University Press, New York, NY.
46. McCabe C and Dixon S, *Testing the Validity of Cost-Effectiveness Models*. Pharmacoeconomics, 2000. 17(5): 501–513.
47. Crnich CJ and Maki DG, *Are antimicrobial-impregnated catheters effective? Don't throw out the baby with the bathwater*. Clin Infect Dis, 2004. 38(9): 1287–92.
48. Frazier AL, et al., *Cost-effectiveness of Screening for Colorectal Cancer in the General Population*. J Am Med Assoc, 2000. 284(15): 1954–1961.

49. Kassirer JP and Angell M, *The journal's policy on cost-effectiveness analyses.* NEJM, 1994. 331(10): 669–670.
50. Drummond MF, et al., *Methods for the Economic Evaluation of Health Care Programmes. Third edition.* 2005, Oxford University Press; Oxford.
51. Philips Z, et al., *Review of guidelines for good practice in decision-analytic modelling in health technology assessment.* Health Technol Assess., 2004. 8(36): 1–158.
52. Briggs A, Claxton K, and Sculpher M, *Decision Modelling for Health Economic Evaluation.* 2006, Oxford University Press; Oxford.
53. Manns BJ, et al., *An economic evaluation of activated protein C treatment for severe sepsis.* N Engl J Med, 2002. 347(13): 993–1000.
54. Chaiyakunapruk N, et al., *Vascular catheter site care: the clinical and economic benefits of chlorhexidine gluconate compared with povidone iodine.* Clin Infect Dis, 2003. 37: 764–771.
55. Marciante KD, et al., *Which antimicrobial impregnated central venous catheter should we use? Modeling the costs and outcomes of antimicrobial catheter use.* Am J Infect Control, 2003. 31: 1–8.
56. Veenstra DL, Saint S, and Sullivan SD, *Cost-effectiveness of antiseptic-impregnated central venous catheters for the prevention of catheter related bloodstream infection.* J Am Med Assoc, 1999. 282(6): 554–60.
57. Claxton K, Sculpher M, and Drummond M, *A rational framework for decision making by the National Institute for Clinical Excellence.* Lancet, 2002. 360: 711–715.
58. Claxton K, et al., *Probabilistic sensitivity analysis for NICE technology assessment: not an optional extra.* Health Econ, 2005. 14: 339–347.
59. Halton K and Graves N, *Economics of preventing catheter-related bloodstream infection.* Emerg Infect Dis, 2007. 13(6): 815–23.
60. Cooper NJ, et al., *Use of evidence in decision models: An appraisal of health technology assessments in the UK since 1997.* J Health Serv Res Policy, 2005. 10(4): 245–250.
61. Coyle D and Lee KM, *Evidence-based Economic Evaluation; how the use of different data sources can impact results, in Evidence Based Health Economics; From effectiveness to efficiency in systematic review,* Donaldson C, Mugford M, and Vale L, Editors. 2002, BMJ Publishing Group: London. 55–66.
62. Harbarth S, Sax H, and Gastmeier P, *The preventable proportion of nosocomial infections: an overview of published reports.* J Hosp Infect, 2003. 54: 258–266.
63. Harris AD, et al., *The use and interpretation of quasi-experimental studies in infectious diseases.* Clin Infect Dis, 2004. 38(11): 1586–1591.
64. Mohan P, Eddama O, and Weisman LE, *Patient isolation measures for infants with candida colonization or infection for preventing or reducing transmission of candida in neonatal units.* Cochrane Database Syst Rev 2007, Issue 3. Art. No.: CD006068. DOI: 10.1002/14651858. CD006068.pub2. 2007.
65. Smaill F and Hofmeyr GJ, *Antibiotic prophylaxis for cesarean section.* Cochrane Database Syst Rev 2002, Issue 3. Art. No.: CD000933. DOI: 10.1002/14651858.CD000933. 2002.
66. Clarke M and Oxman AD, *The Cochrane Reviewers Handbook 4.1.6.* 2003, The Cochrane Collaboration; Oxford.
67. Ramritu P, et al., *A systematic review comparing the relative effectiveness of antimicrobial-coated catheters in intensive care units.* Am J Infect Control, 2008. 36(2): 104–17.
68. Mulrow CD, *Rationale for systematic reviews.* BMJ, 1994. 309: 597–9.
69. Egger M and Smith GD, *Meta-analysis Potentials and promise.* BMJ, 1997. 315(7119): 1371–4.
70. Egger M, Smith GD, and Phillips AN, *Meta-analysis: principles and procedures.* BMJ, 1997. 315(7121): 1533–7.
71. Davey Smith G, Egger M, and Phillips AN, *Meta-analysis Beyond the grand mean.* BMJ, 1997. 315(7122): 1610–4.
72. Egger M and Smith GD, *Bias in location and selection of studies.* BMJ, 1998. 316(7124): 61–6.
73. Egger M, Schneider M, and Davey Smith G, *Spurious precision? Meta-analysis of observational studies.* BMJ, 1998. 316(7125): 140–4.

74. Davey Smith G and Egger M, *Meta-analysis Unresolved issues and future developments.* BMJ, 1998. 316(7126): 221–5.

75. Roberts RR, et al., *Distribution of fixed vs variable costs of hospital care.* J Am Med Assoc, 1999. 281(7): 644–649.

76. Plowman RP, et al., *The Socioeconomic Burden of Hospital Acquired Infection.* 2000, Public Health Laboratory Service; London.

77. Graves N, Halton K, and Robertus L, *Economic costs of health care associated infections, in Reducing harm to patients through healthcare associated infection: the role of surveillance.*, A.C.o.S.a.Q.i.H. Care, Editor. 2008, Australian Commission on Safety and Quality in Health Care: Sydney.

78. Graves N, et al., *The effect of healthcare-acquired infection on length of hospital stay and cost.* ICHE, 2007. 28: 280–92.

79. McGowan JE, *Cost and benefit – a critical issue for hospital infection control.* Am J Infect Control, 1982. 10(3): 100–108.

80. Freeman J, and McGowan JE, Jr, *Methodologic issues in hospital epidemiology. III. Investigating the modifying effects of time and severity of underlying illness on estimates of cost of nosocomial infection.* Rev Infect Dis, 1984. 6(3): 285–300.

81. Haley RW, et al., *Estimating the extra charges and prolongation of hospitalization due to nosocomial infections: A comparison of methods.* J Infect Dis, 1980. 141(2): 248–257.

82. Wakefield DS, et al., *Use of the appropriateness evaluation protocol for estimating the incremental costs associated with nosocomial infections.* Med Care, 1987. 25(6): 481–8.

83. Gertman PM and Restuccia JD, *The appropriateness evaluation protocol: A technique for assessing unnecessary days of hospital care.* Medical Care, 1981. 19: 855.

84. Rishpon S, Lubasch S, and Epstein LM, *Reliability of a method of determining the necessity of hospitalization days in Israel.* Medical Care, 1986. 24: 279.

85. Samore M and Harbarth S, CHAPTER 93. *A Methodologically Focused Review of the Literature in Hospital Epidemiology and Infection Control, in Hospital Epidemiology and Infection Control,* Mayhall CG, Editor. 2004, Lippincott Williams & Wilkins: Philadelphia, PA.

86. Graves N, et al., *Two methods for attributing length of stay to healthcare acquired infection.* Healthcare Infect, 2008. 13: 111–119.

87. Katz MH, *Multivariable Analysis: A Primer for Readers of Medical Research.* Ann Intern Med, 2003. 138: 644–650.

88. Graves N, Weinhold D, and Roberts JAR, *Correcting for bias when estimating the cost of hospital acquired infection: An analysis of lower respiratory tract infections in non-surgical patients.* Health Econ, 2005. 14(7): 755–761.

89. Barnett A and Graves N, *Competing risks models and time-dependent covariates.* Critical Care, 2008. 12: 134.

90. Beyersmann J, et al., *Use of multistate models to assess prolongation of intensive care unit stay due to nosocomial infection.* Infect Control Hosp Epidemiol., 2006. 27(5): 493–9.

91. Spelman D, *Hospital-acquired infections.* Med J Aust, 2002. 176: 286–291.

92. Clec'h C, et al., *Does catheter-associated urinary tract infection increase mortality in critically ill patients.* Infect Control Hospital Epidemiol, 2007. 28(12): 1367–73.

93. Jarvis W, *Selected aspects of the socioeconomic impact of nosocomial infections: morbidity, mortality, cost and prevention.* Infect Control Hospital Epidemiol, 1996. 17(8): 552–7.

94. Klevens RM, et al., *Estimating Health Care-Associated Infections and Deaths in U.S. Hospitals, 2002.* Public Health Rep., 2007. 122(2): 160–6.

95. Peng MM, Kurtz S, and Johannes RS, *Adverse outcomes from hospital-acquired infection in Pennsylvania cannot be attributed to increased risk on admission.* Am J Medical Qual, 2006. 21(Supplement 6): 17S–28S.

96. Brazier J, et al., *A review of the use of health status measures in economic evaluation.* Health Technol Assess, 1999. 3(9).

97. Torrance GW, *Measurement of health state utilities for economic appraisal: a review.* J Health Econ, 1986. 5: 1–30.

98. Geffers C, et al., *The relationship between methodological trial quality and the effects of impregnated central venous catheters.* Intensive Care Medicine, 2003. 29(3): 403–9.

99. McConnell SA, Gubbins PO, and Anaissie EJ, *Do antimicrobial-impregnated central venous catheters prevent catheter-related bloodstream infection.* Clin Infect Dis, 2003. 37(1): 65–72.

100. Ramritu P, et al., *A systematic review comparing the relative effectiveness of antimicrobial-coated catheters in intensive care units.* Am J Infect Control, 2008. 36(2): 104–117.

101. Veenstra DL, et al., *Efficacy of antiseptic-impregnated central venous catheters in preventing catheter-related bloodstream infection: a meta-analysis.* JAMA, 1999. 281: 261–267.

102. Centers for Disease Control and Prevention, *Guidelines for the prevention of intravascular catheter-related infections.* MMWR; Morbidity and mortality weekly report, 2002. 51(RR-10): 1–29.

103. National Institute for Clinical Excellence, *Guide to the Methods of Technology Appraisal.* 2004, London: NICE.

104. Gold MR, et al., *Cost-Effectiveness in Health and Medicine.* 1996, Oxford University Press, New York, NY.

105. Blot SI, et al., *Clinical and economic outcomes in critically ill patients with nosocomial catheter-related bloodstream infections.* Clin Infect Dis, 2005. 41(11): 1591–1598.

106. Warren DK, et al., *Attributable cost of catheter-associated bloodstream infections among intensive care patients in a nonteaching hospital.* Crit care Med, 2006. 34(8): 2084–2089.

107. Martin J, et al., *Intensive Care Resources & Activity: Australia & New Zealand 2003–2005.* 2006, ANZICS, Melbourne.

108. Williams TA, et al., *Data linkage enables evaluation of long-term survival after intensive care.* Anaesthesia and Intensive Care, 2006. 34(3): 307–315.

109. Australian Institute of Health and Welfare, *Australia's Health 2006. AIHW cat. no. AUS 73.* 2006, AIHW, Canberra.

110. Cuthbertson BH, et al., *Quality of life before and after intensive care.* Anaesthesia, 2005. 60: 332–339.

111. Hawthorne G and Osborne R, *Population norms and meaningful differences for the Assessment of Quality of Life (AQoL) measure.* Aust N Z J of Public Health, 2005. 29(2): 136–142.

112. Rechner IJ, and Lipman J, *The costs of caring for patients in a tertiary referral Australian Intensive Care Unit.* Anaesth Intensive Care, 2005. 33(4): 477–482.

113. Graves N, Birrell FA, and Whitby M, *Modeling the economic losses from pressure ulcers among hospitalised patients in Australia.* Wound Repair Regen, 2005. 13(5): 462–467.

114. Braithwaite RS, Roberts MS, and Justice AC, *Incorporating quality of evidence into decision analytic modeling.* Ann Intern Med, 2007. 146(2): 133–141.

115. Harris AD, Lautenbach E, and Perencevich E, *A systematic review of quasi-experimental study designs in the fields of infection control and antibiotic resistance.* Clinical Infectious Diseases, 2005. 41: 77–82.

116. Mermel LA, *Prevention of intravascular catheter-related infections.* Annals of Internal Medicine, 2000. 132(5): 391–402.

117. Morton AP, et al., *Surveillance of healthcare-acquired infections in Queensland, Australia: data and lessons from the first 5 years.* Infect Control Hosp Epidemiol, 2008. 29(8): 695–701.

118. VICNISS, *VICNISS Hospital Acquired Infection Project. Year 5 report – September 2007.* 2007, Victorian Government Department of Human Services: Melbourne.

119. Rechner IJ and Lipman J, *The costs of caring for patients in a tertiary referral Australian Intensive Care Unit.* Anaesth Intensive Care, 2005. 33(4): 477–82.

120. Hawthorne G, Richardson J, and Day NA, *A comparison of the Assessment of Quality of Life (AQoL) with four other generic utility instruments.* Ann Med, 2001. 33(5): 358–370.

121. Manns BJ, et al., *An economic evaluation of activated protein C treatment for severe sepsis.* N Engl J Med, 2002. 347: 993–1000.

122. *Centers for Medicare & Medicaid Services. Medicare Program: Changes to the hospital inpatient prospective payment systems and fiscal year 2009 rates; payments for graduate medical education in certain emergency situations; changes to disclosure of physician ownership in hospitals and physical self-referral rules; updates to the long-term care prospective*

payment system; updates to certain IPPS-excluded hospitals; and collection of information regarding financial relationships between hospitals; final rule.. Federal Register, 2008 (Aug 19). 73(161): 48434–49083.

123. Persson U, Persson M, and Malchau H, *The economics of preventing revisions in total hip replacement.* Acta Orthopaedica Scandinavica, 1999. 70: 163–9.

124. Zell BL and Goldmann DA, *Healthcare-associated infection and antimicrobial resistance: moving beyond description to prevention.* Infect Control Hosp Epidemiol, 2007. 28: 261–264.

125. Cooper BS, et al., *Systematic review of isolation policies in the hospital management of methicillin-resistant Staphylococcus aureus: a review of the literature with epidemiological and economic modelling.* Health Technol Assess, 2003. 7(39): 1–194.

126. Graves N, and McGowan JE, *Nosocomial infection the deficit reduction act and incentives for hospitals.* JAMA, 2008. 300(14): 1577–1579.

127. Burke JP, *Infection control – a problem for patient safety.* N Engl J Medicine, 2003. 348(7): 651–657.

128. Laxminarayan R, *Battling Resistance to Antibiotics and Pesticides: An Economic Approach.* 2003, Resources for the Future; Washington, DC.

129. Laxminarayan R, et al., *Extending the Cure. Policy Responses to the Growing Threat of Antibiotic Resistance.* 2007, Resources for the Future; Washington, DC.

130. Laxminarayan R and Brown GM, *Economics of Antibiotic Resistance: A Theory of Optimal Use.* J Environ Econ Manage, 2001. 42(2): 183–206.

131. Hardin G, *The Tragedy of the Commons.* Science, 1968. 162(3859): 1243–1248.

132. Clements A, et al., *Overcrowding and understaffing in modern healthcare systems: Key determinants in MRSA transmission.* Lancet Infect Dis, 2008. 8(7): 427–34.

133. Graves N, et al., Two methods for attributing length of stay to healthcare acquired infection. Healthcare Infections., 2008. 13: p. 111-119.

Index

Printed in the United Kingdom by
Lightning Source UK Ltd., Milton Keynes
140064UK00002B/100/P